MW00914786

# MASTERING REFLEXOLOGY: REFLEXOLOGY TECHNIQUES TO RELIEVE STRESS AND ANXIETY, THE BENEFITS OF REFLEXOLOGY ON YOUR OVERALL HEALTH AND WELLNESS

D. Beck

D. BECK

Copyright © 2024 D. Beck

All rights reserved

The characters and events portrayed in this book are fictitious. Any similarity to real persons, living or dead, is coincidental and not intended by the author.

No part of this book may be reproduced, or stored in a retrieval system, or transmitted in any form or by any means, electronic, mechanical, photocopying, recording, or otherwise, without express written permission of the publisher.

Cover design by: Art Painter
Library of Congress Control Number: 2018675309
Printed in the United States of America

*I Want to thank you and congratulate you for buying my book*
*Mastering Reflexology: Reflexology Techniques to Relieve Stress and Anxiety, The Benefits of Reflexology on Your Overall Health and Wellness*

# CONTENTS

# INTRODUCTION

Reflexology, also referred to as zone therapy, is an alternative medical practice involving the application of pressure to specific points on the feet, hands, or ears. This pressure is believed to have a positive impact on the person's health and well-being by stimulating corresponding areas in the body. Developed in the early 20th century, reflexology is rooted in the premise that these body parts are connected to certain organs and body systems. Those who practice reflexology assert that it can alleviate anxiety, stimulate nerve function, increase circulation and promote a deep state of relaxation.

Reflexology is often used to address a wide range of ailments and conditions, from headaches and migraines to chronic pain. While this practice is not intended as a replacement for traditional medical care, it can serve as an additional form of therapy in certain cases. Many people find that reflexology helps them cope with the side effects of medical treatments, such as chemotherapy and radiation. Through this holistic approach to health, practitioners of reflexology seek to treat the entire person – body, mind and spirit.

In addition to providing relief from physical discomfort, reflexology can also be used as a form of preventative care. Regular sessions can help strengthen the body's natural defences against illness and disease, making it easier for individuals to maintain good health. By stimulating the nervous system and increasing circulation, reflexology can help reduce stress and improve overall well-being. For this reason, it is often used in conjunction with other forms of self-care such as yoga and meditation.

Hello, it´s me, D. Beck. Before you start reading my book I would like to ask you a favour: If you enjoy reading the book can you please leave an honest review for me in Amazon? - it will mean a lot to me! Thanks in advantage, and now be ready to learn how to master reflexology :)

# CHAPTER 1: WHAT IS REFLEXOLOGY?

Reflexology, sometimes referred to as zone therapy or acupressure massage, is a form of alternative medicine which utilizes the application of pressure to particular points on the feet, hands and ears to produce beneficial effects in other parts of the body. Reflexologists believe that these points correspond with specific organs and systems in the body and that stimulating them can help restore balance to the body and encourage healing.

Reflexology is based on the idea that all areas of the body are connected and can be affected by stimulating certain points. During a reflexology session, practitioners focus on stimulating the reflexes in these areas to encourage relaxation and balance in other parts of the body.

The practice of reflexology is said to have been around since ancient times and is still widely practiced today. It is believed to be beneficial for a wide range of conditions, from headaches and muscle aches to digestive disorders. Reflexology can also be used to reduce stress and improve overall well-being.

## History Of Reflexology

Reflexology is a type of alternative or

complementary medicine that dates back to ancient Egypt. The practice was thought to have originated in China and India, but it wasn't until the late 1800s when an American doctor named William Fitzgerald introduced the concept of reflex zones in the body. He divided the body into ten different vertical zones, each encompassing a different part of the body.

He believed that applying pressure to certain areas of the body would be beneficial in treating illnesses and ailments. He published his theory in a book called Zone Therapy, which was widely accepted as an effective form of therapy for many years.

Since then, several variations of reflexology have been developed including Ingham's Method, introduced in the 1930s. Ingham's method is a system of mapping reflex points on the feet and hands that correspond to various organs and systems throughout the body.

Reflexology has been used for centuries to treat many conditions such as headaches, stress, insomnia, digestive issues, joint pain, and even fertility problems. It's believed that by stimulating certain points in the body, healing energy can be released and restored.

Recent studies have shown that reflexology can help to reduce stress and anxiety while also relieving pain and tension in the body. It has been found to boost immunity, improve circulation, reduce fatigue, and soothe inflammation.

When practiced regularly, reflexology is a wonderful way to promote overall well-being and help you feel more connected to your body. It's a gentle, non-invasive therapy that is suitable for people of all ages and can be used in combination with other treatments or medications for maximum relief.

### Ancient Cultures' Understanding Of Reflexology

It is believed that reflexology has been around for hundreds of years, and many ancient cultures practiced it in some form. The earliest recorded use of the practice is from Egypt, where images of people working on feet have been found dating back to 2330 B.C. It was also mentioned in Chinese medical literature from around the same time period. Other cultures such as Native American and Aboriginal Australians also have a long history of using reflexology.

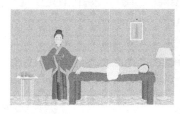

In traditional Chinese medicine, the practice of reflexology is known as "zheng gu" or "acupuncture without needles". In this form of treatment, practitioners would use their thumbs to apply pressure to specific points on the feet and hands in order to stimulate healing energy throughout the body.

In Japan, a form of reflexology called Shiatsu is still practiced today. This type of therapy involves the use of finger pressure to massage certain areas of the body in order to promote healing and relaxation. It is believed that this technique works by stimulating the body's natural energy pathways or "meridians".

Reflexology has also been mentioned in ancient Indian texts such as the Ayurveda and the Charaka Samhita. In both of these texts, reflexology is described as a method of treatment that can help restore balance to the body's energy systems and remove blockages.

Regardless of its origins, it is clear that reflexology has been used for centuries in different cultures all over the world. It is a safe and effective way to treat various health conditions, improve overall well-being, and reduce stress. With the help of modern science, this ancient healing practice can now be utilized by anyone looking for holistic healing methods.

Modern scientists have been able to prove the benefits of reflexology through clinical studies that show how pressure applied to specific areas on the feet and hands can affect the body's internal organs and systems. This has opened up a whole new area of research, which is aimed at understanding how reflexology can be used to treat a variety of ailments.

By harnessing the ancient wisdom of traditional healing methods, such as reflexology, modern medicine is now able to provide more effective treatments for many different health conditions. These treatments can help to reduce stress, improve overall well-being, and even reduce the risk of certain illnesses. As this practice continues to gain traction in modern society, it is important to remember its rich history and understand how powerful an ancient healing method can be.

Reflexology has been found to be especially helpful for treating chronic pain conditions such as fibromyalgia, migraine headaches, and plantar fasciitis. It can also be used to reduce stress levels, improve circulation, and even promote better sleep. As more people learn about the many benefits of this ancient healing method, they will continue to seek out its calming and therapeutic effects for their own health and well-being.

Reflexology is an ancient practice, and its history is filled with stories of healing and wellness. As more people learn about the benefits that it can offer, they will continue to use this unique form of therapy to improve their overall health and well-being. With modern science backing up the age-old wisdom of reflexology, its popularity is sure to only grow in the years to come.

**Reflexology Benefits**

Reflexology is an ancient healing technique that works on the principle of applying pressure to specific points and areas on your feet, hands, or ears. This helps to stimulate the body's natural healing process, as well as provide relief from physical and emotional stress.

The benefits of reflexology are numerous. It can help improve circulation, reduce pain, and relieve stress. It can also help the body to heal itself by improving the function of all systems. In addition, reflexology can improve digestion, regulate hormones, and help balance energy levels in the body.

Reflexology can also be used as complementary therapy for other treatments such as massage or acupuncture. It can provide a gentle, relaxing experience and is often used to reduce anxiety and promote relaxation.

It can also be beneficial for those with chronic pain, including headaches, backaches, and arthritis. Reflexology can help reduce inflammation that is associated with these conditions by stimulating the body's natural healing process.

Reflexology can also be useful in alleviating symptoms of depression, insomnia, and digestive issues. Many people find that reflexology can help reduce stress levels and improve moods.

In addition to these benefits, reflexology may

also help with the prevention of certain diseases by helping the body maintain balance and homeostasis. This in turn can lead to a stronger immune system, improved mental health, and increased overall well-being.

Overall, reflexology is a safe, non-invasive therapy that can provide numerous health benefits. It is best to consult with a qualified reflexologist before beginning any type of treatment. With the help of a trained practitioner, you can find out how reflexology can specifically benefit you.

## The Holistic Approach

The holistic approach to reflexology is based on the belief that when a person's body, mind and spirit are integrated, they can achieve physical, mental and emotional well-being. This means that each part of the individual should be taken into consideration when treating their ailment or illness. Reflexology focuses on stimulating specific areas of the foot or hand to affect corresponding parts of the body and to help restore the natural flow of energy in the body. Treatments can be done with a combination of massage, stretching and pressure on certain areas. By having an understanding of how reflexology works, practitioners can provide their clients with customized treatments that are tailored to their needs. This approach also encourages clients to take responsibility for their own health and well-being by engaging in relaxation techniques such as yoga or meditation. Reflexology can be used in conjunction with other holistic therapies to achieve a greater sense of balance and well-being. With regular sessions, reflexologists strive to help their clients become more in tune with their bodies and minds while also feeling connected to the world around them.

At its core, reflexology is about restoring balance and harmony within the body. Through gentle and precise techniques such as massage, stretching, and pressure on certain areas of the feet or hands, practitioners work to stimulate the body's own healing process in order to achieve balance and well-being. Reflexology is beneficial for a wide range of physical ailments and can also help with emotional issues such as stress and anxiety. Practitioners believe that each individual is unique and tailored treatments should be provided to address their specific needs. With regular reflexology sessions, clients can feel more connected to their bodies as well as the world around them in order to achieve physical, mental and emotional balance.

**How Does Reflexology Work**

Reflexology is an alternative healing therapy that involves applying pressure to specific points on the feet and hands. The theory behind reflexology is that these pressure points correspond to organs and systems in the body. When areas of the foot or hand are stimulated, it can have a positive effect on other parts of the body throughout the body's energy pathways.

When a therapist applies pressure to certain areas of the feet or hands, it can help relieve stress and tension in the body. It is said to promote relaxation and healing throughout the entire body. Reflexology can be used to treat a wide range of physical issues including headaches, joint pain, digestive problems, sinus congestion, asthma and more.

In addition to physical benefits, reflexology is also said to have psychological and emotional effects. The application of pressure to certain points in the feet is thought to release endorphins (the body's natural painkiller) which could lead to an overall sense of well-being, relaxation and calm.

Numerous studies support the benefits of reflexology. It has been used to successfully treat a variety of medical conditions, including fibromyalgia, chronic fatigue syndrome and even cancer. Reflexology is an increasingly popular form of complementary therapy that is gaining recognition from healthcare professionals around the world.

### The Aims And Indications Of Reflexology

Reflexology is a form of alternative medicine that involves applying pressure to specific points on the body in order to produce a therapeutic effect. It is based on the idea that certain areas of the body correspond with other parts, organs and systems within the body. Reflexologists believe that by stimulating these reflex points they can help improve overall health and wellbeing.

The main aims of reflexology are to reduce stress, promote relaxation and improve physical function. It is also believed to have the ability to help with other conditions such as anxiety, depression, headaches and chronic pain.

Reflexology is most commonly used as a means of relaxation but it can be used to target specific areas of discomfort or health issues. When used in conjunction with medical treatment, reflexology can help to reduce the symptoms of certain medical conditions. It is also believed that reflexology has the potential to improve circulation, reduce inflammation and boost the immune system.

Reflexologists may use techniques such as kneading, stroking and squeezing to stimulate reflex points on either feet or hands. They may also use tools such as wooden sticks, stones and crystals to further target these points. Additionally, reflexologists may apply pressure to areas of the body that are not directly connected to a particular organ or system in order to influence healing throughout the entire body.

## Total Relaxation

Total relaxation is the aim of reflexology, and it usually occurs within minutes of beginning treatment. Reflexology can be used to treat many conditions - including headaches, stress, muscle pain, back pain, digestive problems, anxiety and insomnia. It is also beneficial for many chronic illnesses such as arthritis, asthma and multiple sclerosis.

The benefits of reflexology extend beyond physical relaxation; it can also help to improve mental health by relaxing the mind and reducing stress. This is achieved through a combination of massage, breathing exercises and Foot Reflexology techniques that promote relaxation and improve circulation.

## Increase Circulation

Reflexology is a type of massage therapy which aims to increase the circulation of blood and lymphatic fluids around the body, as well as relax muscles in order to reduce stress. It works by stimulating specific points on the feet or hands that correspond with other areas of the body. By applying pressure to these reflex points, practitioners can help achieve improved balance throughout the body. Reflexology is especially beneficial for people dealing with chronic pain, as it can help to reduce inflammation and promote healing by stimulating the body's natural healing mechanisms.

## Helps With The Effective Removal Of Toxins

Reflexology is a healing practice that is growing in popularity as more people look for ways to support their health and well-being. The soothing touch of reflexology helps the body to relax, allowing toxins to be released from the system, resulting in improved overall health. Reflexology massage focuses on specific reflex points throughout the body, stimulating nerve endings, improving circulation and relieving tension. Reflexology has been used to address a range of health issues, including headaches, back pain, fatigue, and digestive problems. It can even be beneficial for those struggling with stress or anxiety.

## Increase Oxygen Levels Within The Bloodstream

Reflexology can also be used to increase oxygen levels within the bloodstream. This is achieved through a combination of massage and Foot Reflexology techniques that stimulate the nerves and promote better circulation. This helps deliver more oxygen-rich blood to the cells in your body, allowing them to function more effectively. With improved circulation, reflexology can help reduce inflammation and improve healing throughout the body.

## Aids The Body To Cleanse Itself Of Toxins

Reflexology aids the body in its natural detoxification processes. By applying pressure to reflex points that align with organs responsible for detoxification - such as the liver, kidneys, and intestines - reflexology can help stimulate these organs into more efficient function. The improved blood circulation and lymphatic flow, brought about by reflexology, also assist in the removal of waste products and toxins from the body. This holistic approach not only cleanses your system, but also supports overall well-being by boosting the immune system, promoting balance, and enhancing your body's natural healing capabilities.

### Aids The Body To Heal Itself

Reflexology is instrumental in aiding the body's inherent healing abilities. It operates on the principle that specific points on the feet and hands are linked to various organs and body systems. When these reflex points are massaged, it stimulates the corresponding body part, invigorating its natural healing processes. This can be particularly beneficial in accelerating recovery from illnesses and injuries, as well as in managing chronic conditions. Moreover, reflexology is known to bolster the immune system, further fortifying the body's defences against diseases. Thus, reflexology is not just a relaxation therapy, but a potent tool for promoting overall health and wellness.

# CHAPTER 2:PRINCIPLES
# OF REFLEXOLOGY

Reflexology is a form of alternative medicine, which involves applying pressure to various parts of the body to promote healing and relaxation. It is based on the idea that certain parts of the body are linked by energy channels (or reflex areas) that correspond with other parts of the body. By stimulating these areas, it is believed that healing and relief from pain can be achieved.

Several principles form the foundation of reflexology, including the concept of energy channels (or "meridians") and the idea that pain and illness can be alleviated by applying pressure to these areas. It is also believed that reflexology may help improve circulation, reduce stress, and enhance overall well-being.

Reflexology is also often used as a form of relaxation. This can involve gently massaging the feet or hands, depending on what areas are being treated. This massage can be customized to address specific needs and ailments. It is believed that by stimulating certain reflex points in the body, it can help reduce pain and improve overall health.

In addition to massage, reflexology can also involve the use of certain herbs and oils. These may be applied to the feet or hands in order to help improve circulation and relax muscles. These remedies can provide an overall sense of relaxation and calmness, while also promoting healing.

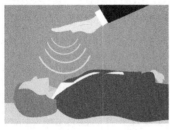

### What Is The Concept Of Energy Flow?

The concept of energy flow in reflexology is based on the idea that all living tissues are comprised of energy pathways connecting to organs in the body. This energetic network can become unbalanced, potentially leading to physical or emotional ailments. By using carefully selected pressure points on the feet and hands, a reflexologist can help to relieve stress and restore balance within this vital network.

Reflexologists believe that the body has an innate ability to heal itself when these energy pathways become blocked or restricted. As a result, they work to unblock and balance these pathways, allowing the body to return to its natural state of well-being. This can be achieved through gentle massage techniques and specific finger pressure applied along reflex points in the hands and feet that correspond to different organs and areas of the body.

Reflexology is also seen as a powerful tool

for strengthening immunity, improving physical performance, reducing pain and aiding in detoxification. It is believed to be especially beneficial for those suffering from chronic fatigue syndrome or irritable bowel syndrome. By focusing on restoring balance within the body's energy pathways, reflexology helps to promote wellness and overall health.

## What Is The Concept Of Energy Channels (Or "Meridians")?

Reflexology is based on the idea of energy channels, or "meridians", which run throughout the body and connect different areas. These energy channels are thought to be filled with a type of life force known as chi that helps promote balance and well-being. In reflexology, it is believed that stimulating certain points along these meridians can help to unblock any built-up chi, improve blood flow, and ultimately restore balance within the body. This is why reflexologists believe that massaging certain points on the hands, feet, and other areas can have a wide range of therapeutic effects. It is believed that this approach can help with a variety of physical and psychological ailments including headaches, digestive issues, and stress. There is also some evidence that reflexology can reduce inflammation, boost the immune system, and even relieve pain. In addition to these therapeutic benefits, many people find that reflexology is simply a relaxing experience.

The gentle massage-like motions of reflexology can help them feel calmer and less stressed.

## The Ancient Chinese Meridians

Reflexology is thought to be based on the principle of ancient Chinese Meridians, which are believed to be pathways through which energy (Qi) flows throughout the body. By using pressure points on the feet, practitioners believe that they can create a balanced flow of energy and restore balance in the body. Reflexology is not just limited to the feet, however; some practitioners also work with pressure points on the hands and ears.

The Chinese Meridians are divided into five major categories: the Lung meridian, Stomach meridian, Gallbladder meridian, Bladder meridian and Kidney meridian. Each of these categories encompasses a number of different pathways which connect to organs in the body. By applying pressure to specific points along these pathways, reflexology practitioners believe that they can stimulate the organs connected to them and restore balance in the body.

## Lung Meridian

The Lung meridian is one of the five major Chinese Meridians and it is associated with the Body's respiration system. It begins at the middle finger on the hand and travels through the tip of the shoulder to connect to several organs, including the lungs, heart, small intestine and large intestine. By stimulating points along this pathway practitioners believe that they can improve the health of the respiratory system and enhance overall well-being.

### Stomach Meridian

The Stomach Meridian is another one of the five major Chinese Meridians and it is associated with digestion and absorption. It starts at the inner corner of the eye and travels down to connect to several organs, including the stomach, spleen, gallbladder and pancreas. By stimulating points along this pathway practitioners believe that they can improve digestive health and promote better absorption of nutrients from food.

### Gallbladder Meridian

The Gallbladder Meridian is another one of the five major Chinese Meridians and it is associated with bile production and detoxification. It begins at the little finger on the hand and travels through the hip to connect to several organs, including the gallbladder, liver, bladder and kidneys. By stimulating points along this pathway practitioners believe that they can improve bile flow and enhance detoxification.

### Bladder Meridian

The Bladder Meridian is one of the five major Chinese Meridians and it is associated with the urinary system. It begins at the outer corner of the eye and travels down to connect to several organs, including the bladder, kidney, small intestine and large intestine. By stimulating points along this pathway practitioners believe that they can improve urinary health and promote better elimination of toxins from the body.

## Kidney Meridian

The Kidney Meridian is one of the five major Chinese Meridians and it is associated with the reproductive system. It starts at the big toe on the foot and travels up to connect to several organs, including the kidneys, adrenal glands, ovaries and uterus. By stimulating points along this pathway practitioners believe that they can improve sexual health and enhance fertility.

## Zone Therapy

Zone Therapy, also known as Reflexology, is an ancient practice that dates back to Ancient Egypt. It involves applying pressure to certain areas on the body in order to stimulate the nervous system and promote healing throughout the body. These points are located on the feet and hands, which correspond with specific organs and systems of the body. By stimulating these points, practitioners believe they can alleviate stress, improve circulation, reduce pain and promote healing.

Zone Therapy is believed to improve the overall health of an individual, as it encourages the body to heal itself. It is based on a holistic approach that promotes balance within the body and helps to restore harmony between mind and body. Practitioners use a variety of techniques during a session, such as massaging, applying pressure to trigger points and other manual therapies.

The benefits of Zone Therapy are far reaching, from improved circulation to reduced stress. It is also said to help improve concentration, increase energy levels and reduce the effects of chronic pain. For those looking for a holistic approach to health and wellbeing, Reflexology may be a great option worth exploring.

Reflexology is often used in conjunction with other treatments, such as massage or acupuncture, in order to maximize its potential benefits. It is important to speak to a qualified practitioner before embarking on any therapy, so that they can ensure it is the right choice for you and tailor the treatment to your individual needs. By understanding how Zone Therapy works and exploring its potential benefits, you can take control of your health and wellbeing.

Another area that Zone Therapy is being used to treat is fertility issues. It has been suggested that by targeting certain areas on the feet, practitioners can improve blood flow to the reproductive organs, helping women get pregnant or dealing with other common infertility issues. If you are struggling with getting pregnant and want to explore alternative options, Zone Therapy is worth considering.

**Maps Of Reflexology**

Maps of reflexology are important tools in understanding how the body is connected and how energy flows throughout it. The chart points on the hands, feet, and ears that correspond to various organs of the body like the heart, lungs, liver, kidneys, etc. By applying pressure at these reflexology points, practitioners can help unblock energy pathways which can promote relaxation and healing.

In some cases, reflexology maps can also be used in tandem with other therapies and treatments. For example, one may use a reflexology map to apply pressure on points that correspond to areas of the body affected by an illness or injury while undergoing physical therapy or chiropractic care. This combination approach can help further facilitate healing and create an overall sense of wellbeing.

Reflexology maps can also be used as part of a meditation practice, as they provide a helpful visual aid for directing breath and energy towards areas of the body that could benefit from healing. By applying pressure to specific reflexology points on the hands, feet, and ears, one can become more mindful of the body and cultivate a greater sense of balance.

Reflexology maps provide an easy way to understand how our bodies are interconnected and how energy flows through them. Understanding these pathways is key in being able to access holistic healing practices that will promote relaxation, wellbeing, and overall health. As more practitioners explore this ancient science, it continues to become an increasingly popular form of alternative therapy.

# CHAPTER 3 : WHAT IS
# REFLEXOLOGY GOOD FOR?

Reflexology is a type of massage therapy that focuses on applying pressure to different points on the feet, hands and ears that correspond to specific parts of the body. It is often used to treat stress-related issues such as tension headaches, insomnia, anxiety, and depression. Reflexology can also help to improve circulation and reduce pain associated with arthritis.

The principles of Reflexology suggest that areas in the hands, feet and ears are linked to particular organs and body systems. Applying pressure to these areas can help restore balance and promote healing throughout the entire body.

Reflexology is believed to have many benefits including: reducing stress, improving sleep quality, boosting circulation, relieving pain, boosting immunity, reducing anxiety and improving mood. Research suggests that Reflexology is an effective alternative treatment for a variety of health issues, including chronic pain, digestive problems and migraines.

Reflexology can be used as both a preventative measure or to help alleviate existing conditions. It may also provide relief from the symptoms associated with certain medical treatments such as chemotherapy and radiation therapy.

## How Reflexology Helps In Improving Mood

Reflexology is becoming increasingly popular as a way to relax and improve mood. It is an ancient practice that has been used in various cultures for centuries and it is now gaining recognition as a valid treatment method for improving overall health and well-being.

Reflexology works by stimulating specific points on the feet, hands, or ears, which are believed to correspond with different organs and systems in the body. By applying pressure on these points, reflexology helps reduce stress and stimulate the body's natural healing abilities. This can have a positive effect on mental health, leading to improved mood and increased energy levels.

Reflexology has been shown to reduce anxiety levels by stimulating relaxation responses in the brain and nervous system. In addition, it can help improve circulation and reduce pain by stimulating the release of endorphins, which are natural hormones that act as a natural painkiller in the body. Reflexology can also be used to treat various physical ailments such as headaches, digestive issues, menstrual cramps, and joint pain.

The benefits of reflexology can be seen in a matter of days. It is important to remember that reflexology works best when combined with other forms of stress-reduction techniques, such as exercise, yoga, meditation, and deep breathing. Consistently practicing these activities will produce the best results for improving overall physical and emotional health.

**Steps For Improving Mood By Reflexology:**

1. Make an appointment with a certified reflexologist.

2. During the, focus on deep breathing and relaxation techniques to maximize the effects of reflexology.

3. Maintain regular appointments with your reflexologist to ensure that you get the maximum benefit from each session.

4. In between sessions, take time for yourself by engaging in activities such as yoga, meditation, or light exercise.

5. If possible, practice self-reflexology at home between appointments. This can be done using a reflexology chart and applying pressure to the points listed on it.

By taking these simple steps and combining them with regular reflexology visits, you will soon experience improved moods and an overall feeling of health and wellbeing. Reflexology is an incredibly powerful tool for restoring balance to the body and mind, making it a great choice for those seeking to improve their mental health.

## How Reflexology Helps In Improving Sleep Quality

Reflexology is an ancient healing technique that involves the use of pressure points on the body to release tension and stress, reduce pain, improve circulation, and promote overall relaxation. It has been used for centuries to help people relax and fall asleep more easily. By massaging specific reflex points on the feet or hands, it helps to stimulate the nervous system and induce a deep state of relaxation. This can lead to improved sleep quality and duration, making it an ideal tool for those suffering from insomnia or other sleeping disorders.

Reflexology is often used in conjunction with other therapies such as massage, aromatherapy or herbal remedies. The massage helps to relax the entire body, while specific reflex points on the feet or hands may be massaged to target specific areas of the body that may be causing stress or tension. Additionally, aromatherapy oils can be used in reflexology as a way to further enhance relaxation and promote peace of mind. Herbal remedies can also be used in combination with reflexology for increased healing benefits.

Reflexology is an excellent tool for improving sleep quality and duration. It can help individuals relax and fall asleep more quickly, and it also helps to decrease stress levels by targeting specific reflex points in the body. Furthermore, when combined with other therapies such as massage, aromatherapy or herbal remedies, the benefits of reflexology are further enhanced.

**Steps For Improving Sleep Quality By Reflexology:**

1. Start with a foot massage: Begin by massaging the feet and working up towards the ankles to relax the muscles and increase circulation. Work in small circular motions on each part of the feet for several minutes until relaxed.

2. Move onto reflexology: Once your feet are relaxed, use thumbs to apply pressure to various reflex points on both feet. These points are connected to various parts of the body, and pressing them will help to stimulate the nervous system and induce relaxation.

3. Use aromatherapy: After you've massaged your feet with reflexology, add a few drops of lavender oil to a cotton ball and lightly rub it on the feet for an extra layer of calming aroma.

4. Finish with a foot massage: Once the reflexology and aromatherapy are done, finish off the session by massaging your feet one more time to further relax them and prepare your body for sleep.

By following these steps, you can use reflexology as an effective way to improve your sleep quality. It helps to relax the body and reduce stress levels, while also promoting better circulation. Additionally, when combined with other therapies such as aromatherapy or massage, reflexology can be an effective tool for improving sleep quality and duration.

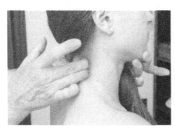

## How Reflexology Helps In Reducing Stress

Reflexology is a form of alternative medicine that has been in practice for centuries. It involves manipulating specific zones or reflex points on the hands, feet and ears to stimulate healing throughout the body. Reflexologists believe that this manipulation helps reduce stress and tension by stimulating the nerves and releasing endorphins.

Recent studies have shown that reflexology can help reduce stress, improve mental clarity and emotional wellbeing. By targeting specific areas of the body that are believed to be linked to stress, reflexologists can help reduce cortisol levels in the body and promote relaxation. Reflexology has also been shown to have a positive effect on the immune system by increasing lymphatic circulation and reducing inflammation.

Reflexology can also help with headaches, neck pain and other physical ailments. The treatment has been found to not only reduce pain but also improve overall health. By stimulating specific reflex points, it can help to regulate the nervous system and balance hormones in the body.

**Steps For Reducing Stress By Reflexology:**

1. Relaxation: The first step of reflexology is to relax the body and mind. Reflexologists use various techniques such as stretching, massage and breathing exercises to create a relaxed, stress-free state.
2. Stimulation: Once the body is relaxed, the reflexologist will begin to stimulate specific points on the hands, feet and ears with the hands, thumbs and fingers.
3. Sensations: As the reflexologist applies pressure, various sensations such as warmth or tingling may be felt by the patient. These sensations indicate that the body is responding to the treatment and releasing tension.
4. Results: After completing a session of reflexology, patients often report feeling relaxed and energized with improved sleep and mood. It is important to have regular sessions in order to maintain the stress-reducing effects of reflexology.

## How Reflexology Helps In Migraines And Headaches

Reflexology is an ancient healing art that has been used for centuries to help alleviate physical and emotional ailments. It is based on the idea that different parts of your body are connected to specific areas of your feet, hands, and ears. By applying pressure to these reflex points, practitioners believe they can stimulate the natural healing energy in the body and improve overall health and wellbeing.

Research suggests that reflexology can be effective in relieving symptoms of migraines and headaches. Studies show that patients who received regular treatments experienced a significant decrease in the severity and frequency of their headaches. They also had improved moods, reduced stress levels, and better quality sleep.

Reflexologists believe that the foot has many nerve endings, which can be stimulated through massage and reflexology to restore the natural balance of energy throughout the body. This in turn helps reduce pain, relax the mind, and improve overall wellbeing. Reflexologists believe that migraines often come from a disruption of energy flow between different parts of the body – for example, an imbalance in hormones or too much stress on the nervous system. By restoring the balance of energy in the body, reflexology can help reduce migraine symptoms and improve overall health.

In addition to relieving head pain, research suggests that reflexology may also have other positive effects for people with migraines. It can help reduce stress, which is a major trigger of headaches, and it can improve circulation throughout the body to promote healing. By stimulating the reflex points in the feet, it can also help restore balance and harmony throughout the body.

## Steps Of Migraines And Headaches By Reflexology:

The first step in the reflexology treatment for migraines and headaches is to identify which areas of the foot are connected to where you are experiencing pain. Reflexologists believe that each point on your feet correlates with a specific organ or area of the body, and by stimulating these points, they can help restore balance and promote healing. The practitioner will then use several techniques to stimulate the reflex points, such as massage and applying pressure with their thumbs or fingers. This is meant to relax your muscles and improve circulation in the area.

The second step of a reflexology treatment for migraines and headaches is to do a postural assessment. The practitioner will take note of any imbalances throughout the body and determine which areas need extra attention. For example, if you are carrying extra tension in your neck and shoulders, the practitioner may focus on those points to help relieve that tension and restore balance throughout the body.

Finally, the practitioner will do a series of stretches and relaxation techniques to further reduce tension and pain. This is meant to give your body time to relax so it can heal itself. The practitioner may also recommend lifestyle changes, such as reducing stress or avoiding trigger foods, to help reduce your risk of future headaches.

While there is no cure-all for migraine and headache relief, reflexology has been proven to be effective in relieving symptoms and improving overall wellbeing. By targeting the body's natural energy pathways and restoring balance throughout the body, reflexology can help reduce pain and discomfort and promote healing.

### How Reflexology Helps In Arthritis Pain

Reflexology is an ancient technique that has been proven to be beneficial in assisting with numerous ailments and conditions, especially arthritis. It works by applying pressure to specific points on the feet or hands as a means of stimulating the body's natural healing processes. Reflexology can help reduce pain and inflammation associated with arthritis, as well as improve circulation and promote relaxation.

While the exact cause of arthritis is unknown, it is believed that this condition is caused by an imbalance in the body's energy field. By manipulating pressure points on the feet and hands in areas where nerve endings are located, reflexology helps restore balance to the body's energy field and promote healing.

The benefits of reflexology for arthritis include:

-Pain relief: Reflexology can help reduce pain and inflammation associated with arthritis. This is because it helps to stimulate blood flow in the affected areas, which helps to relieve stiffness and tightness.

-Improved circulation: By stimulating circulation throughout the body, reflexology not only helps to reduce swelling but also improve overall health and wellness. Improved circulation means more oxygen and nutrients can be delivered to the cells, which helps reduce pain.

-Promotes relaxation: Reflexology is also known for its calming effects. By massaging pressure points in the feet and hands, reflexology helps to relax the body and mind. This relaxation can help improve sleep quality, and ultimately lead to better overall health.

**Steps Of Arthritis Pain By Reflexology:**

1. Start by consulting a qualified reflexologist. They will assess the areas of your feet and hands that require attention, as well as any other symptoms you may be experiencing and suggest an appropriate treatment plan for you.
2. During the session, the reflexologist will use their fingers to massage pressure points in the feet or hands. This helps to stimulate the body's natural healing processes and can help reduce pain associated with arthritis.
3. The reflexologist will also use various techniques such as kneading, pressing, and rubbing to further promote relaxation.
4. Reflexology should be done on a regular basis for best results. Depending on your individual situation, this may mean weekly or monthly sessions.

Reflexology is a safe and natural way to help reduce pain and inflammation associated with arthritis and other conditions. It can be a great complement to your traditional medical care, helping you find relief from your symptoms without the use of medications or surgery. If you're looking for an alternative way to manage your arthritis, consider giving reflexology a try. Not only can it help reduce your pain, but it can also improve your quality of life and promote relaxation.

## How Reflexology Helps In Chronic Pain

Reflexology is a powerful form of alternative healing that has been used for centuries to provide relief from chronic pain and other ailments. This ancient technique uses pressure points in the hands, feet, ears, and face to stimulate the body's natural self-healing mechanisms. It works by targeting specific areas in order to reduce inflammation, improve circulation and restore balance to the body.

The hands and feet are the most common reflexology points, as they contain a large number of nerve endings and pressure points that correspond to different organs and muscles in the body. By applying pressure on these areas, reflexologists can help relieve tension, improve circulation, reduce inflammation and promote healing. It is also believed that reflexology can help to reduce stress and anxiety, improve sleep quality, and boost energy levels.

Reflexology can be an effective treatment for chronic pain sufferers. It has been shown to reduce inflammation in the body, which can help to relieve pain in muscles and joints. This type of therapy can also stimulate the release of endorphins, which are natural pain-relieving hormones. Additionally, reflexology can help to release toxins and improve circulation, which can further relieve the pain associated with chronic conditions.

While reflexology cannot cure chronic pain conditions, it can certainly be an effective way of managing the symptoms. By targeting specific pressure points in the hands and feet, sufferers can find relief from their aches and pains. It is also important to note that reflexology should be used in combination with other treatments, such as medications and physical therapy, for maximum effectiveness.

**Steps Of Chronic Pain By Reflexology**

1. Find the right reflexologist: The first step in using reflexology to treat chronic pain is to find a qualified and experienced reflexologist who can help you manage your symptoms.
2. Identify problem areas: Once you have chosen a suitable practitioner, they will be able to identify which points are causing the most discomfort and should be targeted during treatment.
3. Recognize the pressure points: The reflexologist will then apply gentle, yet firm pressure to the specific areas to stimulate them and reduce inflammation.
4. Re-balance energy flow: During a session, the reflexologist will aim to restore balance in your body's energy flow by

releasing tension and unlocking blocked pathways.

5. Take regular breaks: It is important to take regular breaks during the session, as too much pressure can lead to further pain and discomfort.

6. Be aware of side effects: Reflexology has been found to have few side effects, however some people may experience slight dizziness or nausea after a session.

7. Make lifestyle changes: As well as undergoing reflexology, it is important to make lifestyle changes such as eating a healthy diet and getting regular exercise in order to achieve long-term relief from chronic pain.

## How Reflexology Helps In Boosting The Immune System

Reflexology is a type of therapy that involves applying pressure to certain points on the body, known as "reflex points." These reflex points are believed to be connected to different organs and systems in the body. The goal of this form of therapy is to help relieve stress and tension, and promote healing in the body. Research has shown that reflexology can help boost the immune system, reduce inflammation, alleviate pain, and improve circulation.

The practice of reflexology is based on the concept

that there are specific points in the body that correspond to different organs and systems. By applying pressure to these reflex points in a precise manner, it is believed that tension can be released and energy pathways opened up, which can help improve overall health and well-being.

When reflexology is used to boost the immune system, it helps enhance the body's natural ability to fight off infection and illness. This is done by stimulating the lymphatic system, which helps remove toxins from the body more efficiently. It also reduces stress levels, as high levels of stress can weaken the immune system.

### Steps Of Boosting The Immune System By Reflexology

The following is a general guideline of the steps involved in boosting immunity with reflexology:

1. Identify the areas that need to be addressed. This includes identifying any areas that may have become congested due to stress or other environmental factors.
2. Use pressure and massage techniques on the identified points, focusing on releasing tension and opening up energy pathways.
3. Stimulate the lymphatic system with gentle massage techniques to help remove toxins from the body more efficiently.

4. Work on any reflex points that are related to organs or systems which play an important role in immunity, such as the colon and digestive system.

## How Reflexology Helps In Fighting Cancer

Reflexology is a complementary therapy that has been used for centuries to help people cope with physical and emotional pain. This ancient practice works by applying massage techniques to various pressure points in the feet, hands and ears. The idea behind reflexology is that these pressure points are linked to different parts of the body, allowing practitioners to target specific body parts or organs.

When it comes to cancer, reflexology can be used to help reduce stress and improve physical wellbeing. Stress is known to have a negative impact on the body's immune system which can make it harder for the body to fight off disease and heal wounds. By reducing stress with reflexology massage, people are able to boost their natural healing capabilities and help their body cope with cancer treatment.

Reflexology can also be used to help manage pain that is associated with cancer, as well as the side effects of chemotherapy or radiation therapy. The massage techniques can be tailored to target various parts of the body, including the areas that are affected by cancer treatments. This helps to reduce inflammation in those areas and promote healing.

Finally, reflexology can also be used to stimulate circulation throughout the body, allowing for better movement of fluid and nutrients throughout the body. This helps promote tissue healing and regeneration which can help people suffering from cancer symptoms.

### Steps Of Fighting Cancer By Reflexology

Reflexology can help people with cancer in many ways, and the following steps are often recommended by experts for those looking to use reflexology as a complementary therapy:

1. First, it is important to speak with a certified reflexologist about your needs and goals for treatment. This will allow the practitioner to tailor the massage techniques to target the areas that are of most concern.
2. When receiving a reflexology massage, focus on deep breathing and relaxation techniques to get the most out of each session. The key is to allow your body to relax and open up so that the massage techniques can be effective.
3. It is important to drink plenty of water before and after each session, as this helps flush out toxins from the body.
4. After your session, take time to listen

to your body and respond accordingly. If you feel any discomfort or pain, let your reflexologist know so they can adjust their techniques accordingly.

5. Finally, be sure to get regular reflexology massage sessions if possible as this helps keep the body in balance and strengthens its healing capabilities.

Reflexology can be an effective complementary therapy for those dealing with cancer, allowing them to reduce stress and manage pain while promoting healing. By speaking with a certified practitioner and following the above steps, those using reflexology can experience the full benefits of this ancient practice.

## How Reflexology Helps In Boosting Fertility

Reflexology has been a popular form of healing for centuries, and it is now being used more than ever to help couples boost their fertility. It is believed that reflexology works by stimulating different parts of the body and improving blood circulation. This encourages the production of hormones which can have a positive impact on conception rates.

The most common areas targeted with reflexology are the feet, hands and ears. Each area holds different points which can be used to stimulate certain organs into action. Applying pressure or massaging these areas can relax and unblock energy pathways, allowing for better circulation within the body.

Reflexology works by improving overall health in many ways: it strengthens the immune system, decreases stress levels and improves the quality of sleep. All these things are beneficial for fertility, as they help to ensure that your body is functioning optimally.

Studies have suggested that reflexology can be particularly helpful in cases of unexplained infertility. It can also provide relief from conditions such as endometriosis and PCOS which may be contributing factors to a couple's difficulty in conceiving.

**Steps Of Boosting Fertility By Reflexology:**

1. Find an experienced reflexologist who is familiar with treating fertility issues.
2. Make sure you communicate any health concerns and lifestyle habits to your specialist, as this will help them determine the best course of treatment for you.
3. During a session, the reflexologist will use their hands to apply pressure to certain areas on your feet, hands and ears. This helps to stimulate the organs associated with fertility.
4. After a session, your reflexologist may

recommend lifestyle changes which will help you get the best results from your treatment. These could include dietary adjustments or exercise routines.

Overall, reflexology is a safe and non-invasive therapy which has been used for centuries to boost fertility. It can be a great complement to other treatments, such as IVF or hormone therapy, and may be able to help couples who are struggling to conceive. If you think reflexology could be the right solution for you, make sure you find an experienced practitioner who is trained in this therapy.

## Correcting Hormonal Imbalances

Reflexology is an excellent way to help correct hormonal imbalances in the body. It works by targeting specific points in your feet and hands, as well as other areas of your body, that are directly connected to the different hormones present in our bodies. When pressure is applied on these reflexes, it stimulates energy pathways which can ultimately lead to the regulation of hormones in our bodies.

Reflexology is also known to help reduce stress, which can be a trigger for hormone imbalances. This happens because when pressure is applied on certain reflex areas it releases endorphins, which are natural feel-good hormones that create a relaxed feeling and lower cortisol levels. This helps to optimize hormonal balance, and in turn, regulate the body's processes.

Another benefit of reflexology is that it can help improve circulation in the body and promote better nutrient absorption. This can also lead to improved hormone production as a result of increased blood flow. Additionally, reflexology encourages lymphatic drainage which helps the body eliminate toxins more effectively, thus optimizing hormone balance as well.

## How Reflexology Helps In Improving Digestion

This therapy works by applying pressure to points on the hands or feet, known as reflex points, which correspond to particular parts of the body. When these reflex points are stimulated they can help stimulate nerve impulses and improve circulation throughout the affected organ systems. By improving circulation in the abdomen, digestive organs can be better nourished and digestion improved.

Moreover, reflexology helps to reduce stress levels in digestion system as well. Stress is a known trigger for many chronic digestive disorders such as Irritable Bowel Syndrome (IBS). By helping to reduce stress levels, reflexology helps release tension that has built up in the body and allows the digestive system to relax and operate more efficiently. It also encourages healthy blood flow which can further improve digestion by carrying essential nutrients throughout the entire body.

Finally, reflexology helps to improve nerve function in the digestive system as well. When these nerves are not functioning properly, they can prevent food from passing through your digestive tract, leading to constipation or indigestion. By stimulating the reflex points, reflexology helps to improve nerve functioning which allows food to move more efficiently through your digestive tract and improves digestion overall.

**Steps Of Improving Digestion By Reflexology:**

1. Identify the reflex points in the feet and hands that correspond to the digestive organs.
2. Apply gentle pressure to these areas, using your thumbs or fingers, for several minutes
3. Move your hands in a circular motion along each area for further stimulation
4. Focus on breathing deeply as you do so, to help relax both mind and body
5. Repeat this process once or twice a day for the best results

Reflexology is a simple yet effective method of improving digestion, by helping to reduce stress levels, improve circulation and nerve functioning. Through regular practice, it can help to keep your digestive system in balance and maintain optimal health!

By increasing blood flow to the digestive organs, reflexology can also help to alleviate bloating and other uncomfortable symptoms of digestive disorders. This is done by helping to improve the communication between the brain and the digestive system, allowing it to respond better to signals from your body.

### How Reflexology Helps In For Nerve Problems

Reflexology is an ancient healing art that has been used for centuries to help treat nerve disorders, relieve pain and reduce inflammation. Reflexology works by stimulating specific points on the feet, hands and ears which correspond with different organs in the body. When these areas are stimulated, it can help improve circulation, reduce stress levels, and boost overall relaxation. Reflexology can be a great option for those dealing with nerve problems, as it can help reduce pain and inflammation, while promoting relaxation and healing.

Reflexology may also be helpful in relieving the symptoms of certain types of neuropathy, such as carpal tunnel syndrome. Reflexology works by stimulating the nerves that run along the length of the arm and hand. This type of therapy can help to reduce inflammation and improve circulation in the affected areas, providing relief from tingling or numbness. In addition, it can help relax the muscles in the hand and arm, which may also alleviate some of the pain associated with carpal tunnel syndrome.

Reflexology is also beneficial for those suffering from sciatica. Sciatica is a nerve condition that causes pain to radiate from the lower back down the leg and into the foot. Reflexology can help to reduce this pain by stimulating specific points along the spine, as well as points on the feet. This type of therapy can help to decrease inflammation, improve circulation and reduce muscle tension in the affected areas.

Finally, reflexology can be beneficial for those dealing with migraines and headaches. By stimulating specific points on the head and neck, reflexology has been shown to reduce pain associated with these conditions. It can also help to improve circulation in the area, which can help to relieve muscle tension that may contribute to migraine symptoms.

**Steps For Nerve Problems By Reflexology:**

1. Start by sitting comfortably in a chair or lying on your back, whichever is more comfortable for you.
2. Take long, slow deep breaths to relax and allow your body to become still.
3. Using the thumb of one hand, gently

massage each foot in turn in circular motions for several minutes at a time. Move up and down the foot, concentrating on any areas that feel tender or sore.

4. Apply firm pressure to specific points of the feet for 30-60 seconds at a time. These points correspond with different organs in the body and by stimulating them can help improve circulation and reduce pain and inflammation caused by nerve problems.

5. To finish, use long, sweeping strokes from the toes to the ankles on both feet. This helps draw out any built up tension and further relax your body.

## How Reflexology Helps In Blood Clots

Reflexology is an alternative therapy that involves the use of pressure points on the hands and feet to stimulate different parts of the body. It has been used for centuries to help people manage pain, reduce stress, and improve overall health. In recent years, researchers have begun to discover how it can also be beneficial for helping with blood clots.

Recent research has found that reflexology can reduce the risk of stroke or heart attack caused by a clot in the arteries. This is because it stimulates circulation and helps keep blood flowing freely throughout the body, which helps prevent clots from forming in the first place.

In addition to helping with blood clots, reflexology has also been found to help improve overall health. It can reduce stress, relieve pain, and improve sleep quality. This is because it stimulates the release of endorphins, which are natural hormones that help promote relaxation and well-being.

Reflexology treatments should be done by a qualified professional in order to maximize its effects. The pressure points used in reflexology have been carefully mapped out and applied to specific areas of the body. It is important to find a practitioner who has experience and expertise in this field, as they will know which points to activate for the best results.

**Steps For Blood Clots By Reflexology:**

1. First, the reflexologist will assess your health and identify any specific areas of concern.
2. During the session, they will apply pressure to various points on your feet or hands that correspond to parts of the body affected by a clot.
3. Depending on the severity of the clot, they may use special techniques such as lymphatic drainage or massage to help

reduce swelling and pain.

4. Finally, they may recommend lifestyle changes such as diet and exercise that will help improve your overall health.

## How Reflexology Helps In Improving General Well-Being

It is based on the principle that certain areas of the body are linked to other parts of the body and can be stimulated by applying pressure to these points. By stimulating certain reflex points, it helps to balance out energy in the body, which in turn leads to improved health and wellness.

Reflexology is a very safe and natural means of healing, as it has no known side effects and it does not involve the use of drugs or surgery. It can be used for many different ailments, including physical pain, stress-related issues, headaches, digestive disorders, insomnia and fatigue.

The process of Reflexology involves the application of gentle pressure to specific points on the feet and hands. By stimulating these reflex points, it helps to reduce tension, improve circulation and promote relaxation in the body. Additionally, it can be used to help manage chronic pain, as well as improving overall balance in the body.

Reflexology is often combined with other holistic practices such as massage, aromatherapy or yoga, as it works synergistically to promote healing and well-being.

## Steps For Improving General Well-Being By Reflexology:

1. Get a professional Reflexology treatment. This is the best way to ensure that you are receiving an accurate and therapeutic massage, as it provides a controlled pressure to the reflex points in order to achieve maximum results.
2. Self-massage the feet and/or hands with oil or lotion before going to bed each night. This helps to relax the body and mind, as well as promoting better circulation.
3. Incorporate yoga or other stress-relieving activities into your routine, in order to promote further relaxation of the body and mind.
4. Invest in comfortable shoes that provide enough support for your feet, as this can help to reduce any tension or pain felt in the feet.
5. Relax and take time for yourself. Stress can have a negative effect on your health, so it is important to try to reduce stress levels in order to improve overall well-being. Taking some time out each day for yourself will help you manage stress and feel more balanced both physically and

mentally.

6. Consider the use of natural remedies such as essential oils to help create a calming atmosphere in your home.
7. Practice mindful breathing techniques to relax and calm your mind, as well as improving the overall flow of energy throughout your body.
8. Eat healthy meals that are full of vitamins and minerals, as this can help with boosting your immune system and provide additional energy for daily activities.
9. Drink plenty of water in order to hydrate and flush toxins from the body, helping you feel more energized and alert.

By following these steps, you can help improve your general well-being with reflexology. This natural form of healing can be an effective means to achieving better overall health, as it helps to balance energy in the body and promote relaxation.

**Multiple Sclerosis**

Reflexology is a great way to help those with multiple sclerosis. This condition affects the central nervous system, which can lead to severe pain and fatigue. Reflexology treatments directly target these areas of the body, helping to relax muscles and reduce inflammation. The practice also helps promote relaxation, which can alleviate stress-related symptoms as well as mental health issues caused by the condition. Studies have also found that reflexology can help reduce chronic pain, aid in neurological function and improve quality of sleep. It can even be used as an alternative form of treatment for those looking to avoid medications. Reflexology is a great tool for anyone living with multiple sclerosis, helping them to feel more relaxed and in better control of their own health.

# CHAPTER 4: FOOT REFLEXOLOGY

Foot Reflexology is a great way to naturally reduce stress and tension in your body. It can also help improve circulation, balance energy levels, detoxify the body, and bring about a sense of relaxation. When you practice Foot Reflexology, you use pressure points on the soles of your feet to relieve tension and promote healing. With regular practice, you can gain a better understanding of how your body works and discover new ways to relieve tension.

Foot Reflexology is a safe and simple practice that anyone can do. All you need is a reflexology chart, which shows the various pressure points on the feet, as well as their corresponding benefits for overall health and wellbeing. It's important to learn how to apply the right amount of pressure to each point, as applying too much pressure can cause discomfort.

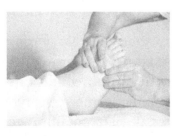

## Basics Of Foot Reflexology

Foot Reflexology is an ancient practice that has been used for centuries to improve overall wellbeing. It uses pressure points on the feet to help reduce stress and tension, increase circulation, and provide relief from pain or other issues. By targeting certain areas of the foot with massage techniques, one can achieve a greater sense of balance in the body and mind.

The main goal of reflexology is to promote balance and harmony by stimulating the body's natural healing mechanisms. This is accomplished by applying specific pressure points on the feet, which correspond to different organs or systems in the body. For example, massaging certain areas of the foot can help reduce stress, improve circulation in a specific area, or aid digestion.

In addition to its healing powers, reflexology can also be used to help people better understand their bodies and how all the parts are connected. By understanding what each pressure point relates to and how it affects overall health, one can become more conscious of the body's needs. This awareness can help create a greater sense of self-care and prevent certain health issues from developing in the first place.

### Effects Of Foot Reflexology On Anxiety And Pain

Some of these studies found that reflexology may be effective for reducing anxiety and providing pain relief, even for those with chronic conditions such as arthritis. Additionally, some research suggests that reflexology may help to improve circulation and stimulate the body's natural healing processes.

For those looking to learn more about foot

reflexology, it is important to know that there are various points on the foot corresponding to different organs and systems in the body. By applying pressure to certain areas, it is possible to target specific parts of the body and provide relief.

For instance, a reflexologist may use their thumbs or fingertips to apply pressure along the medial area of the foot, which corresponds with the inner organs of the body. Through this pressure, a trained reflexologist can help to relieve tension and provide respite from physical discomfort.

In addition to helping manage anxiety and pain levels, reflexology can also be beneficial for mental health in general. Studies have shown that it may be effective for calming the mind, reducing stress, and improving overall wellbeing.

At the end of a session, it is important to take some time to relax and unwind. Taking a hot bath or enjoying a massage can further help the body to assimilate the effects of reflexology.

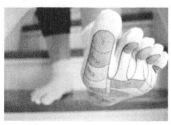

### Foot Reflexology Chart

Foot Reflexology Chart is a tool that has been used for centuries to provide relief to those who are suffering from various ailments and discomforts. This chart provides a visual representation of the body's pressure points, which are connected to different organs and bodily functions. Through foot reflexology, it is possible to find relief from pain and discomfort in any area of the body.

By stimulating the pressure points in the feet, it is possible to alleviate symptoms associated with organ imbalances. This can help to improve overall health and well-being by bringing balance back to the body. Foot reflexology may also be used to promote relaxation and reduce stress levels.

In addition to using a foot reflexology chart as an aid for relief, it can also be used to identify potential health issues in the body. By analyzing the pressure points in the feet, it may be possible to identify any areas of imbalances or inflammation in other parts of the body. This could allow for early diagnosis and treatment of conditions before they become more severe.

Foot reflexology is becoming increasingly popular due to its ability to offer holistic relief and its potential for diagnosing health issues. It is important, however, to consult with a qualified professional in order to ensure that the techniques used are safe and effective. With proper guidance, reflexology can be an invaluable tool for maintaining good health.

## Ailments

Foot reflexology is often used to help manage a range of ailments. Commonly, it is utilized to relieve symptoms of stress, anxiety, and sleep disorders. It's also shown efficacy in dealing with chronic conditions such as migraines, sinusitis, and digestive issues. Furthermore, reflexology has been reported to assist with pain management for conditions such as arthritis and back pain. However, it's crucial to remember that while foot reflexology can provide relief and aid in the management of these conditions, it should not replace professional medical advice and treatment. Always consult with a healthcare provider for serious or persistent health concerns.

**Discomforts**

Discomforts can manifest as physical symptoms like pain, stiffness, or inflammation, or as emotional symptoms such as stress, anxiety, or depression. Reflexology, particularly foot reflexology, can play a significant role in managing these discomforts. The technique involves applying specific pressure to reflex points on the feet, which correspond to different organs and parts of the body. By doing so, it can help in alleviating a range of discomforts. However, it's important to understand that reflexology does not cure these conditions but assists in managing the symptoms and improving quality of life. Much like other complementary therapies, it's best used in conjunction with traditional medical treatments and under the guidance of a professional.

**Pain Management**

Reflexology is not only a deeply relaxing experience, but can also be used as an effective tool for pain management. Research has found that targeting specific reflex points on the feet can help to reduce levels of chronic pain and improve quality of life. By stimulating nerve endings on the feet, pressure can be applied to certain areas of the body in order to promote healing and provide relief from pain and tension.

Reflexology not only works on the feet but can be used to treat other areas of the body as well. Areas such as the hands, ears, and even face can benefit from reflexology techniques. By applying pressure to specific points in these areas, practitioners are able to bring about relaxation and reduce levels of stress or chronic pain in different areas of the body.

The benefits of reflexology are not just limited to pain management however. Many people report feeling more energized and refreshed after a reflexology session, along with improved digestion and better sleep quality. In addition, regular reflexology treatments can help to boost immunity and reduce stress levels.

### Eyestrain

Foot reflexology can also be used to help alleviate the symptoms of eyestrain. Symptoms of eyestrain can include headaches, blurred vision, dry eyes, and soreness or redness in the eye area. Reflexology helps reduce stress which can trigger these symptoms by stimulating specific points on the feet that correspond with certain areas of the body - including those associated with the eyes. It can also help increase circulation to the eyes, improving oxygenation and reducing inflammation. Foot reflexology is a natural way to reduce eyestrain and bring relief to tired eyes. Reflexologists around the world recommend this technique as an effective way to relieve stress and tension from eyestrain-related symptoms. It can be used in combination with other treatments or as a preventative measure to keep your eyes healthy and strong. Reflexology is an easy and safe way to stay on top of eyestrain-related issues, and may even help you get ahead of any potential problems in the future.

**Pressure Points In The Foot For Reflexology**

Reflexology is an ancient practice that uses the pressure points in your feet to promote the healing of the body. By stimulating certain areas of the foot with massage and reflexology techniques, it is believed that these pressure points can help relieve pain and improve circulation throughout the body.

The pressure points are located on both sides of each foot, and there are seven main areas known as the reflex zones. Each of these points corresponds to a different organ or body part, and when stimulated through massage or pressure, it is believed to have a healing effect on that area.

The big toe represents the head and brain, while the next toe indicates the eyes and ears. The ball of the foot relates to the chest and lungs, while the arch of the foot is related to the stomach and intestines. The heel corresponds to the spine, lower back and kidneys area.

The two pressure points at the base of each toe correspond to the liver and bladder, respectively. Finally, there are two points in between each toe which link up with your reproductive organs.

**Top Of The Toes:**

The tops of the toes each contain a pressure point that is believed to correspond to various parts of your neck, face and mouth. When these points are stimulated it is said to be beneficial in alleviating sinus pain and congestion.

**Middle Of The Toes:**

The middle of the toes contains pressure points that are said to correspond to the heart muscle and circulation. Stimulating these points can help promote good blood flow throughout the body and alleviate issues such as high blood pressure, chest pain and fatigue.

**Bottom Of The Toes:**

The bottom of the toes contains pressure points that relate to the gall bladder and stomach.

Stimulating these points is believed to help with digestion and alleviate indigestion, constipation and bloating.

**The Base Of The Pinky Toe:**

The base of the pinky toe is a pressure point that corresponds to the spleen and its ability to filter toxins from the body. Stimulating this point can help improve immunity and also reduce stress levels.

**The Outer Lateral Side Of The Foot:**

The outer lateral side of the foot is home to pressure points that are believed to connect with the liver. Stimulating these points can help detoxify and cleanse your body, as well as improve energy levels.

**The Outer Medial Side Of The Foot:**

The outer medial side of the foot contains pressure points that are related to your body's ability to absorb nutrients and eliminate waste. Stimulating these points is believed to help with digestion and nutrient absorption, as well as reduce bloating and constipation.

**The Lateral Side Of The Ankle:**

The lateral side of the ankle contains pressure points that are believed to connect with your adrenal glands. Stimulating these points is said to help reduce stress levels and improve energy levels.

**The Medial Side Of The Ankle:**

The medial side of the ankle is home to pressure points that are said to correspond to your kidneys and their ability to filter toxins from the body. Stimulating these points can help improve detoxification, reduce inflammation and promote healthy kidney function.

**Middle Of The Top Of The Foot:**

The middle of the top of the foot contains pressure points that are believed to link up with your endocrine system. Stimulating these points can help reduce stress levels, improve energy levels and regulate hormones.

**Warnings/Contraindications**

Reflexology should not be used on individuals with open wounds, infectious diseases, or any type of skin disorder. Additionally, it is contraindicated for people who have had recent surgery or suffer from arteriosclerosis and thromboses. Reflexology is also not the most suitable remedy to use during pregnancy as it can stimulate contractions in the uterus and cause miscarriage.

Before a reflexology session, the therapist must know of any health conditions or medications you are taking to ensure they can take this into account during the treatment. Reflexology should not replace medical advice and consultation with your doctor regarding any medical condition.

Finally, if at any time during the treatment, you feel uncomfortable or have any kind of pain, be sure to tell the therapist so they can adjust their technique accordingly.

Reflexology is a great way to relax and experience a different form of therapeutic massage - just make sure you are aware of the potential warnings and contraindications beforehand.

**How To Prepare For A Foot Reflexology Session**

A foot reflexology session can be an incredibly relaxing and rejuvenating experience. To ensure you get the most out of your session, there are a few easy steps to follow.

First, make sure you're wearing comfortable clothing that won't be too constricting during the massage. Loose-fitting clothes are the best option.

Second, you'll want to make sure your feet are clean and free of any dirt or debris. This will help increase circulation during the massage and allow your reflexologist to work more effectively.

Third, it's important to drink plenty of water both before and after your session. This will keep your body hydrated and help flush out toxins that are released during the massage.

Fourth, make sure you arrive early so you can relax

before your session begins. This will give you a chance to discuss any concerns or questions with your practitioner, as well as help ensure there won't be any time pressure during the session itself.

Finally, if possible, find a quiet place to rest after your session. Your body may need time to adjust to the massage and this time of rest can be incredibly beneficial for your wellbeing.

**Finger Walking**

In finger walking, the practitioner applies pressure to certain points on the feet and hands with their thumbs or fingers. The pressure helps stimulate blood flow and relax tense muscles in the foot, which can be beneficial for reducing pain and promoting full-body relaxation. Finger walking can also help reduce stress, improve circulation, promote relaxation of the joints, and help release toxins from the body.

To perform finger walking correctly, start by standing with your feet flat on the floor. Grasp one foot in both hands and begin to massage the bottom of that foot, using your thumbs or fingertips to apply pressure. Work up along the arch of the foot and then down through the heel. Move slowly across all the points on the bottom of the foot, applying pressure as you go.

Once you've massaged both feet with finger walking, move on your hands. Again, start near the base of the thumb and massage up along it until you reach the wrist. Repeat this motion with all ten fingers to ensure that all areas are receiving appropriate amounts of pressure.

**Foot Soaking**

Another important part of preparing for a reflexology session is foot soaking. Foot soaking helps soften calluses and cleans the feet, while also promoting relaxation of the muscles in the feet and lower legs. To start, fill a basin or tub with warm water and add Epsom salts or essential oils if desired for extra relaxation benefits. Place your feet into the warm water and allow them to soak for at least 10 minutes.

Once you've finished soaking your feet, gently pat them dry with a towel and inspect the soles of your feet for any areas that may need extra attention during the session. If there are any calluses or thick patches of skin on the soles of your feet, use a pumice stone or exfoliating scrub to help soften and remove them.

By following the steps outlined above, you can ensure that your reflexology session is as beneficial as possible. Taking the time to prepare each step of the way will help maximize your relaxation experience and reap all of the potential health benefits that reflexology has to offer.

**Foot Balm Application**

Once you have prepared your feet with finger walking and soaking, it is recommended to apply a moisturizing foot balm or cream. This will help condition the skin on the soles of the feet and ensure that you feel relaxed and comfortable throughout your reflexology session. Choose a product that is specifically designed for use on feet, as some products can contain harsh ingredients that can further irritate the skin.

This step is especially important if you have sensitive skin on the soles of your feet, as applying the foot balm can help reduce any potential irritation or discomfort that may occur during your session.

These steps will help ensure a successful reflexology session and allow for maximum benefit from it after it's over. Taking care to follow the steps and properly preparing the feet before a session can make all the difference in its effectiveness.

**Breathing Exercises**

Before beginning your reflexology session, it is important to engage in deep breathing exercises. This will help you relax and mentally prepare yourself for the upcoming massage. Start by sitting or lying down in a comfortable position and closing your eyes. Then, take a few deep breaths in and out through your nose, allowing your stomach to expand with each inhalation and deflate on the exhalations. As you continue to focus on your breathing, allow any tension or worries to melt away with each exhale.

# CHAPTER 5: HANDS REFLEXOLOGY

Hands Reflexology is a traditional form of Asian massage that has been used to promote healing and relaxation for centuries. It involves the use of pressure points on the hands, feet, and ears to massage away tension and stimulate circulation.

By applying pressure in specific areas of the hand, reflexologists can help to alleviate pain, reduce stress, improve circulation, and even promote healing. This type of massage can also be used as a preventative measure, working to keep the body in balance and functioning optimally.

Hands Reflexology is best performed by experienced practitioners who understand the underlying principles and anatomy of reflexology. Practitioners must use gentle pressure when applying pressure to points on the hand, avoiding any discomfort or pain. It is also important to take time to listen to the patient's needs, so that each session of reflexology can be tailored specifically for them.

In Hands Reflexology, practitioners use techniques such as thumb walking and kneading to stimulate pressure points on the hands. Specialized tools may also be used in some cases, such as small wooden rods, plastic cups, or metal tools.

Depending on the patient's needs and what is being treated, the reflexologist may focus on certain points more than others. Generally speaking, though, all of the major pressure points are usually worked into each session.

**What Are The Basics Of Hands Reflexology?**

1. It is believed that reflexology works by stimulating the body's natural healing response. The idea is that each point on your hands corresponds to a certain area of the body – for example, any reflex points in the palms correspond with the chest and lungs, while points at the base of the thumb relate to digestion.

2. When pressure is applied to these points, many therapists believe it helps relieve stress and tension in the body's organs. This is thought to improve circulation, stimulate healing, and improve overall health.

3. Reflexology is typically administered using circular strokes with either the thumbs or fingers on both hands at once. The therapist will apply gentle pressure for a few minutes at each point before moving on to the next one.

4. While reflexology is not a medical treatment, some people have found it to be beneficial for relieving stress and

tension. People with chronic pain or other conditions may find that regular treatments help alleviate their symptoms and improve their quality of life.

5. Reflexology is often used in conjunction with other relaxation techniques such as massage or aromatherapy. It is important to consult with a qualified reflexologist before beginning any treatment, as they can provide personalized advice and help tailor an individualized plan that works best for you.

6. Whether it's used on its own or in conjunction with other treatments, hand reflexology can be a valuable tool for promoting overall well-being. By focusing on the specific points on your hands, you can help to relax and relieve tension in key areas of the body.

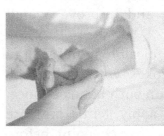

### Benefits of Hand Reflexology

Hand reflexology is growing in popularity as a way to help reduce stress, improve circulation, and promote healing throughout the body. By applying pressure to specific points on the hands, practitioners can relieve tension and improve overall health. Here are just a few of the benefits of hand reflexology:

**Reduced Stress**

Hand reflexology has been found to reduce stress and anxiety in patients. In a study published by the National Institutes of Health (NIH), participants were given 10-minute hand reflexology sessions twice a week for 3 weeks. At the end of the study, participants reported feeling less stressed than they had before starting the treatment. This indicates that regular hand reflexology can have a positive effect on stress levels.

In addition to reducing stress, hand reflexology can also be beneficial for pain relief. In the same study published by NIH, participants reported feeling less pain after receiving hand reflexology treatments. This suggests that regular hand reflexology may help reduce chronic pain symptoms as well.

The benefits of hand reflexology go beyond just physical effects. It can also be beneficial for mental health. In one study, participants who received hand reflexology treatments reported feeling less depressed and anxious than those who did not receive the treatments. This suggests that hand reflexology may help to improve mood and reduce mental health symptoms.

**Improved Circulation**

Hand reflexology can also help to improve circulation throughout the body. By applying pressure to specific points on the hands, practitioners are able to stimulate blood flow and increase oxygen delivery to cells throughout the body. This can help to reduce fatigue and improve overall physical performance.

In addition, improved circulation may help to flush out toxins from your body. When circulation is poor, toxins can accumulate in the body and lead to a variety of health problems. Improved circulation can help to remove these toxins from your body, leading to better overall health.

**Relief Of Pain And Discomfort**

Hand reflexology can also be used to relieve pain and discomfort throughout the body. By applying pressure to specific points on the hands, practitioners can help to reduce tension and improve the functioning of the body's organs. This can be helpful for people suffering from chronic pain conditions such as fibromyalgia, arthritis, and back pain.

In addition to reducing pain, hand reflexology can help to improve joint mobility. By manipulating certain points on the hands, practitioners are able to stimulate the release of endorphins which can help to reduce inflammation and improve joint range of motion.

**Improved Digestive Health**

Hand reflexology can also be beneficial for your

digestive system. By stimulating specific points on the hands, practitioners are able to stimulate the release of enzymes which can help to break down food more effectively. This can lead to improved absorption of nutrients from food, leading to better overall health.

In addition to improving digestion, hand reflexology can also help to reduce constipation and bloating. By stimulating the digestive system, practitioners are able to improve the functioning of the intestines, helping them to move food more efficiently through the body. This can lead to fewer gastrointestinal symptoms like constipation and bloating.

**Clearer Skin**

The increased circulation that results from hand reflexology can help to flush out toxins in the body, leading to clearer skin and fewer breakouts. By improving circulation, practitioners are able to speed up the process of detoxification which helps to remove impurities from your cells. This can lead to improved cell functioning and fewer skin problems like acne and wrinkles.

**Increased Immunity**

Finally, hand reflexology can help to boost your immune system. By stimulating certain points on the hands, practitioners are able to stimulate the lymphatic system which is responsible for fighting off infections and illnesses. This can help to keep your body healthy and reduce your risk of getting sick.

Overall, hand reflexology has many benefits that go beyond just reducing stress and pain. With regular treatments, practitioners can help to improve circulation, digestive health, skin clarity, and immunity. This range of benefits makes hand reflexology an excellent choice for anyone looking to improve their overall health.

**Hands Reflexology Chart**

The Hands Reflexology Chart is a tool which helps understand the relationship between the hands and their reflex points in the body. It can be used to identify areas of tension or stress, as well as pinpoint where pressure should be applied for maximum benefit. The chart divides the hand into four sections: thumb, index finger, middle finger and little finger. Each section includes several points that correspond to different parts of the body, from the head and neck down to the feet.

When using the chart, it's important to remember that each reflex point corresponds to a particular area of the body. Applying pressure on these points can help reduce tension and stress in those areas. Additionally, applying pressure on some points may also increase circulation in other parts of your body.

## Pressure Points In The Hand For Reflexology

Reflexology is a natural healing method that uses pressure points in the hands to treat various physical and emotional ailments. It may be used to reduce pain, alleviate stress, improve circulation, and even help with digestion. By gently manipulating certain areas of the hand, therapists can stimulate healing energy pathways throughout the body.

### Palm

The palm of the hand is an area with many reflex points that correspond to different parts of the body. By pressing these reflex points, it can help stimulate and balance energy in the body. This type of reflexology is known as palm or digital reflexology.

This technique works by applying pressure to specific points on both hands, usually at the same time. By constantly pressing on these reflex points, the body's energy can be released and redirected which can help improve overall health and wellness.

For example, pressing on points in the palm of your hand that correspond to your brain can help reduce headaches and mental stress. Likewise, pressing on points related to the digestive system can help improve digestion and prevent constipation.

Reflexology can be used as an effective treatment for many different ailments and conditions, and by applying constant pressure to reflex points in the palm of your hand you can help reduce symptoms associated with these conditions.

## Thumb

The thumb plays a significant role in hand reflexology as it contains several important pressure points. Different areas of the thumb correspond to various parts of the body, including the lungs and the brain. Applying pressure on the base of the thumb can help alleviate respiratory issues while pressing the tip of the thumb can aid in mitigating headaches and stress. The thumb is often manipulated during reflexology sessions for its versatility and accessibility. By incorporating thumb pressure points into a reflexology routine, one can further enhance the benefits of this holistic healing technique.

## Fingers

The fingers, much like the thumb, hold a wealth of pressure points that correspond to different organs and body parts in reflexology.

- **Index finger:** The index finger is related to the stomach and the colon. Applying pressure to the tip of the index finger may alleviate digestive issues and improve gut health.
- **Middle finger:** This finger corresponds

to the heart, small intestine, and circulation. Pressure applied here could help with cardiovascular health and blood flow.

- **Ring finger:** Reflexologists associate the ring finger with the lungs and respiratory system. By applying pressure to this finger, one may find relief from breathing problems and allergies.
- **Pinky finger:** The smallest finger represents the kidneys, head, and neck. Pressing on its tip might aid in mitigating headaches, neck pain, or kidney-related issues.

Understanding and utilizing these pressure points can significantly increase the effectiveness of your reflexology sessions, providing a comprehensive treatment that addresses multiple areas of the body.

**Wrists**

The wrists contain reflex points that can be used to relieve tension in the upper body. By gently massaging these areas of the wrist, it can help relax tense muscles and reduce pain or discomfort caused by chronic inflammation or injury. This type of reflexology can also aid in relieving stress and anxiety associated with work or other life stresses.

**Arms**

The arms also have pressure points that can be

used to relieve strain in the shoulders, elbows, and wrists. Massaging these areas can help improve the range of motion and reduce stiffness. This technique may be used for athletes who experience tightness in the arms due to repetitive use or exercise-induced injury.

## Warnings/Contraindications

Practitioners of certain reflexology techniques must be aware of the contraindications and warnings for this type of therapy. Researching potential health concerns and complications is key before beginning any form of reflexology treatment.

Individuals with a known history or risk of high blood pressure, heart disease, diabetes, glaucoma, thrombosis, or nerve damage should always be informed and consulted by a doctor before beginning reflexology treatments.

Reflexology is not recommended for individuals who are pregnant, have recently had surgery or experience chronic pain. Reflexology should also be avoided if an individual has an active infection or inflammation in the feet. If any of these conditions exist, please contact your physician before beginning reflexology treatments.

It is important to understand that while reflexology may help reduce stress and tension, it is not intended to diagnose or treat any medical condition. If you are experiencing pain or discomfort, please contact your doctor right away. Reflexologists cannot diagnose, prescribe medications, or perform any invasive techniques.

Finally, although the vast majority of reflexology treatments are generally safe and comfortable, there may be certain areas of the feet that are too sensitive to touch. If this happens, please inform your practitioner immediately so they can adjust their approach accordingly.

# CHAPTER 6: EAR REFLEXOLOGY
# AND FACIAL REFLEXOLOGY

Ear reflexology is a powerful and holistic healing technique that uses pressure points located in the ears. By stimulating these reflex points, it can help promote relaxation, reduce pain, improve circulation, and even alleviate some symptoms of chronic illnesses. Ear reflexology has become increasingly popular among those looking for an alternative health treatment, or simply to improve their overall health and wellbeing.

The theory behind ear reflexology is that the body is divided into several zones and each part of the ear corresponds to different areas in the body. By gently stimulating these points, practitioners are able to help release tension and balance energy flow throughout the body.

**Benefits of Ear Reflexology**

1. Stress Relief: Ear reflexology is known to be an effective and natural way to relieve stress. The gentle stimulation of the reflexology points in the ear can help promote relaxation and release tension, allowing you to feel more relaxed and balanced.

2. Improved Sleep Quality: Stimulating the reflexology points located in the ear

can also help improve sleep quality. By promoting relaxation and calming the mind, it can help relieve insomnia as well as reduce fatigue.

3. Pain Relief: Ear reflexology has been used to effectively treat a number of different types of pain including headaches, neck pain, and shoulder pain. By stimulating specific points in the ear related to these areas, it can be an effective way to reduce discomfort and promote relaxation.

4. Boosts Immunity: By stimulating the reflexology points located in the ear, it can help improve your body's immune system and reduce inflammation. Stimulating these points can also help to balance hormones and promote better overall health and well-being.

5. Improved Circulation: Ear reflexology is known to be an effective way to increase blood flow throughout the body. Stimulating these points can help to promote better circulation and reduce the risk of developing certain illnesses and health conditions.

**Ear Reflexology Chart**

The Ear Reflexology chart is a great tool for understanding how to use reflex points located in the ear to provide relief and healing. It can be used both as an instructional guide and as a reference.

The chart consists of several illustrations that identify specific areas of the ear, including the outer, middle, inner ear and even the brainstem. Each illustration shows the reflex points, along with their corresponding physical effects when stimulated.

For example, stimulating the outer ear can help alleviate headaches, sinus congestion and neck pain. The middle ear is known to be linked to providing relief for digestive issues, while the inner ear can provide relief from colds and coughs. Finally, the brainstem is associated with feelings of relaxation and calmness.

By using the Ear Reflexology chart, practitioners can quickly identify which reflex points to focus on in order to provide relief from a wide variety of ailments. It is also helpful for locating other areas that may need attention, such as those related to emotional well-being. Ultimately, this chart provides an effective way to practice reflexology in order to promote overall health and wellness.

## Pressure Points In The Ear For Reflexology

Reflexology is a form of alternative medicine that involves massaging or applying pressure to specific points on the body in order to promote healing and relaxation. Ear reflexology, specifically, uses massage techniques along certain points in the ear that are thought to correspond with other parts of the body.

## Helix

The helix is the larger outer ridge of the ear and can be used to massage for many different benefits. It is connected to the kidney, bladder, liver and gallbladder, which are all important bodily organs that should function optimally in order to maintain good health. Massaging this area can help improve circulation, reduce inflammation and improve overall organ functioning.

## Antihelix

The antihelix is the inner ridge of the ear and is thought to be associated with the spleen, stomach and pancreas. This area can be massaged to help improve digestion as well as reduce inflammation. It can also help to reduce stress and anxiety levels which are often connected to digestive issues.

## Tragus

The tragus is the small pointed lobe at the front of the ear and is thought to be connected to the throat and thyroid gland. Massaging this area can help with neck pain, sore throat, and even headaches. It may also help regulate hormones that are related to the thyroid gland.

## Anti-Tragus

The anti-tragus is the area of the ear opposite the tragus, and it is linked with reproductive organs including the ovaries and testes as well as hormones. Massaging this area can help to relieve menstrual cramps, reduce PMS symptoms, and improve fertility. It may also help to regulate hormones that are associated with these organs.

## Crus Of Helix

The crus of the helix is located at the base of the ear and connects to the heart, circulatory system and lymphatic system. Massaging this area can help to improve circulation, reduce inflammation, and promote relaxation. It can also help to reduce stress levels which can be beneficial for overall cardiovascular health.

## Concha

The concha is the bowl-shaped part of the ear and corresponds to the respiratory system, as well as the heart. Massaging this area can help to improve breathing, reduce congestion, and even ease asthma symptoms. It may also help to reduce stress levels which can be beneficial for overall respiratory health.

## Lobule

The lobule connects with digestion, kidneys and adrenal glands. Massaging this area can help with digestion issues such as constipation or bloating, as well as reduce inflammation in the kidneys. It may also help to regulate hormones that are associated with these organs.

By using reflexology on the ear, it is possible to experience many potential health benefits such as improved organ functioning, reduced stress levels, and improved overall well-being. Learning the proper massage techniques for each specific area of the ear is important in order to experience these benefits safely and effectively.

## Warnings/Contraindications

Reflexology is generally considered a safe practice for most people, but certain contraindications should be taken into consideration. Those who have recently had surgery, have circulatory issues, nerve damage and/or diabetes should always consult their doctor prior to beginning reflexology treatments to ensure it is the right therapy for them. People with active cancer, pain disorders, high fever or active infections should also consult their doctor before proceeding. Additionally, pregnant women should always check with their physician prior to beginning reflexology as certain points may be contraindicated due to the risk of premature labor and miscarriage.

Reflexology is not recommended for people with pacemakers or those who use aids such as hearing aids, since the pressure used may affect their functioning. Additionally, people with metal plates, pins or other implanted devices should consult their doctor since these could be affected by the pressure applied during treatment.

Before beginning a reflexology session, it is important to inform your therapist about any medical conditions you may have so that they can make sure that the treatments are tailored to fit your needs. It is also important to speak up if any pressure applied during the session feels too intense or causes discomfort, as this will help ensure a safe and successful treatment session.

Finally, it should be noted that reflexology does not take the place of traditional medical treatments - only a qualified doctor can diagnose and treat illnesses and conditions. As such, reflexology should always be used in conjunction with medical advice, not as a substitute.

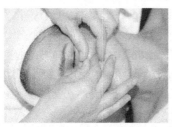

### Facial Reflexology

Facial Reflexology is a relaxing and deeply effective treatment that can help to reduce stress, improve circulation, and restore balance within the body. With specialized techniques that stimulate reflex points on the face, neck, and scalp, Facial Reflexology helps to unblock energy pathways in the body and promote healing from within.

The treatment begins with a consultation in order to understand the client's issues and needs. During the treatment, gentle pressure is applied to certain points on the face, neck, and scalp which correspond with areas of the body. The practitioner will use their knowledge of Chinese medicinal massage techniques (Tui Na) as well as other modalities such as acupressure and lymphatic drainage to create a customized treatment that addresses the individual's needs.

**Benefits Of Facial Reflexology**

Facial Reflexology is a form of healing that can be used to help alleviate physical, mental and emotional health issues. It's been used in ancient cultures for centuries, yet only recently has it become more popular with modern medical practitioners due to its many potential health benefits.

1. Improved Circulation: Facial Reflexology helps to improve circulation in the face, which in turn can help brighten and give an overall healthy glow to your complexion.
2. Stress Relief: It is believed that facial reflexology can help relieve stress and tension, possibly due to its calming effect on the nervous system. This could make it helpful for people who suffer from anxiety or depression.
3. Reduced Pain: It's possible to use facial reflexology as a form of pain management for certain conditions, such as headaches and migraines. This is because it works

to relax the facial muscles which can help reduce tension-related pain.

4. Improved Immune System: Facial Reflexology has been found to improve the immune system by stimulating lymphatic drainage. This can help the body to better filter toxins and waste, as well as allow it to absorb vital nutrients.

5. Better Sleep: As mentioned previously, Facial Reflexology helps to reduce stress and tension which can have a positive effect on sleep quality. It's thought that this type of reflexology could be beneficial for those who suffer from insomnia or other sleep disorders.

Overall, Facial Reflexology can be a helpful tool for maintaining physical and emotional well-being. It can help to reduce stress, improve circulation, and provide relief from certain types of pain. Additionally, it may even be beneficial for boosting the immune system and improving sleep quality. For these reasons, many people turn to this type of healing therapy as an alternative or complement to conventional medicine.

**Pressure Points In The Facial For Reflexology**

Facial reflexology is a gentle touch therapy that uses pressure points on the face to promote relaxation and healing. It can be used for a variety of ailments including headaches, migraines, sinus

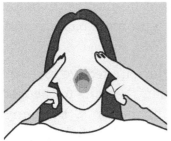

problems, stress, and even facial wrinkles. This type of therapy can help restore balance and release tension in your body.

**The Third Eye**

Point is the most important point to use in facial reflexology. It is believed that this pressure point helps unblock energy channels and restore balance in the body. When done correctly, facial reflexology can provide a great sense of relaxation and improved well-being.

**The Temporal Point**

The Temporal Point is the second most important point in facial reflexology. It is connected to the brain and helps reduce headaches, migraines, and tension in the neck.

**The Jaw Point**

The Jaw Point is useful for reducing stress and tension in the jaw area as well as alleviating TMJ, facial wrinkles, and sinus problems. The Chin Point also helps reduce soreness in the lips and chin area.

**The Top Of The Head Point**

This point can be used to relax the mind and body,

as well as reduce stress and headaches. It helps open up energy channels to promote balance and restore well-being.

Facial reflexology is a gentle yet effective form of therapy that can provide many benefits for people suffering from a variety of ailments. By using the correct pressure points, you can help reduce stress and tension in your body while promoting relaxation and improved well-being. Reflexology is non-invasive and can be done at home or in a professional setting. With regular reflexology sessions, you may experience increased energy levels, improved sleep, and even smoother skin.

**Warnings/Contraindications**

Reflexology should not be used by:

- Those with a fever or inflammation.
- For any individual who has recently undergone surgery, there can be serious complications and interactions.
- Individuals with cancer, heart disease, high blood pressure, diabetes, or any other medical condition without consulting their doctor first.
- Pregnant women should only use reflexology after consulting their physician.
- Those who have had a stroke or other neurological disorder should not try reflexology.

Additionally, it's important to note that facial

reflexology is not meant to replace traditional medical treatments and should only be used in conjunction with the advice of a trained professional. Be sure to discuss any health concerns you may have with your doctor before engaging in any type of reflexology.

It is also wise to avoid using facial reflexology on the face if you are prone to getting headaches or experiencing migraines. If this is the case, it's best to seek out a trained professional who has experience dealing with these types of issues.

## Auriculotherapy

Auriculotherapy is an ancient and natural healing modality that dates back thousands of years. It utilizes the auricle, or outer ear, as a map of the entire body. By applying pressure or stimulation on specific points in the outer ear, practitioners can target different areas of the body for treatment. This technique can be used to treat various conditions, including pain and stress, as well as hormonal imbalances. It is also believed to be able to stimulate the body's own healing processes.

Auriculotherapy has been found to help treat a wide variety of conditions and ailments. This technique can be used to help with headaches, chronic fatigue, digestive issues, menstrual dysfunctions, and even addiction. Auriculotherapy can also help to balance hormones and improve moods. It is an effective way to treat physical pain, as well as emotional issues such as stress, anxiety, and depression.

## Benefits Of Auriculotherapy

Auriculotherapy includes a reduction in pain, increased relaxation, and improved overall health. This technique can also be used to reduce stress levels and improve sleep quality. Auriculotherapy is a non-invasive treatment with few side effects, making it an excellent option for those seeking natural healing solutions. With continued use, patients may experience long-lasting relief from their symptoms.

## How It Works

Auriculotherapy uses a range of stimuli such as electrical stimulation, magnets, and massage to target specific points on the ear. These ear points are thought to correspond to other parts of the body, allowing practitioners to address health issues in those areas. By stimulating these points, it is believed that energy blockages can be released and healing can occur.

Auriculotherapy is often combined with other healing modalities such as acupuncture, massage therapy, and biofeedback. This allows practitioners to further address the root cause of an issue in order to promote overall health and wellness. Auriculotherapy has also been found to be beneficial in treating a range of psychological issues, including anxiety, addiction, and depression.

## Electrical Stimulation

Auriculotherapy also uses electrical stimulation to target specific points in the ear. This method involves using an electrical device that emits a small current. The patient may feel mild sensations during this process, but it is generally painless and non-invasive. Electrical stimulation is thought to help relieve tension in the body and promote healing by increasing blood flow to affected areas.

Auriculotherapy can be performed by a variety of practitioners, including acupuncturists, naturopaths, chiropractors, and massage therapists. Before beginning treatment, it is important to consult with a health professional who is familiar with this technique in order to ensure that the patient receives the best possible care. With continued use, auriculotherapy may provide positive, long-term results for those seeking natural healing solutions.

### Magnets

Magnets are also used in auriculotherapy. This method involves placing small, magnetic beads on specific points of the ear. The magnets then apply mild stimulation to these parts of the body, believed to help reduce pain and tension. Magnets can be worn continuously for long periods of time or removed after each session. Although this technique is generally considered safe, it is important to consult with a health professional beforehand in order to ensure that the magnets are the right size and type for your condition.

## Massage To Target Specific Points On The Ear

Massage can also be used in auriculotherapy to target specific points on the ear. This method involves gently massaging these areas with firm pressure in order to stimulate healing and reduce tension. Massage can be beneficial for those suffering from pain, stress, or fatigue. It is important to consult with a health professional before beginning this technique as they may have specific instructions on how to perform the massage. With continued use, massage can help improve overall health and well-being.

## Pressure Points In The Auriculotherapy

Auriculotherapy utilizes pressure points in the ear as a way to target different areas of the body. Each part of the ear has been mapped out to correspond with certain organs and systems in the body. By applying stimulation or pressure at these points, practitioners can address conditions related to those parts of the body.

There are a few different types of pressure points

that are commonly used in auriculotherapy. These include acupressure and trigger points. Acupressure involves using firm pressure on specific points of the ear to release energy blockages and promote healing. Reflexology utilizes gentle pressure to stimulate reflex areas throughout the body. Trigger points involve further pressing into specific parts of the ear in order to create localized changes.

**Acupressure**

Acupressure is a type of auriculotherapy that involves applying firm pressure to specific points on the ear. This technique is believed to help open up energy pathways and unblock areas where there may be tension or pain. It is also thought to improve circulation in the body, helping to flush out toxins and promote healing. Acupressure is generally painless and has few side effects, making it an excellent option for those seeking natural healing solutions.

**Trigger Points**

Trigger points are another type of auriculotherapy that involves applying more pressure to specific areas of the ear. This technique is believed to be useful in targeting localized issues such as headaches, neck pain, and muscle tension. It is important to consult with a health professional before beginning this technique as they may have specific instructions for how much pressure should be applied.

## Warnings/Contraindications

Auriculotherapy is generally considered a safe and non-invasive treatment. However, it is important to consult with a health professional beforehand in order to determine if this technique is right for you. The following persons should generally avoid auriculotherapy:

- Those with pacemakers, metal implants, or other medical devices
- Pregnant women
- Persons with active bleeding or infection in the ear area
- Persons with extreme sensitivity to touch or pressure

It is also important to note that there is limited scientific evidence to support the effectiveness of auriculotherapy. As with any medical treatment, it is important to consult with a qualified health professional before beginning.

# CHAPTER 7: WHAT ARE
# REFLEXOLOGY TECHNIQUES?

Gua sha therapy

Gua sha therapy is an ancient Chinese healing technique that uses a special tool to press and scrape the skin in order to stimulate circulation and release tension. It is believed to help relieve chronic pain, reduce inflammation, improve immunity, and soothe emotional stress. By stimulating the meridians and energy pathways (or "qi") of the body, Gua sha can also help to balance the body's energies and bring greater physical, mental, and emotional well-being.

In addition to its healing effects on physical health, Gua sha is also thought to be beneficial for spiritual development. According to traditional Chinese medicine, the practice of using special tools to press and scrape the skin helps open up blocked energy pathways in the body. This, in turn, can help to balance the flow of qi and promote greater spiritual awareness.

Not only is Gua sha an effective way to improve physical health, but it also has other benefits including improved sleep quality, better emotional wellbeing, improved mental clarity, and more. It is a safe and natural healing modality that can be used by anyone who is looking to improve their health and well-being. With the right technique and tools, it can be a powerful tool for cultivating health and harmony in body, mind, and spirit.

Gua sha therapy does not require any special equipment or techniques, but it is important to learn how to use the tools correctly in order to get the most benefit from the practice.

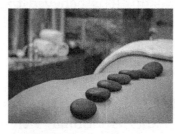

### The Tools

The most common tools used in Gua sha therapy are jade and other stones that have been carved into curved shapes. They are typically either flat or spoon-shaped, with rounded edges to help reduce the risk of skin irritation. The stones should be smooth and free of any sharp points or edges. Other tools, such as ceramic spoons, wooden paddles, and special comb-like knives, can also be used.

When using jade or other stones during Gua sha therapy, it is important to use light and steady pressure. The tool should be moved in gentle strokes up the body from the bottom to the top. As you move the stone, it should leave behind a redness that will fade after an hour or so. This redness indicates that the Gua sha technique has been effective in stimulating circulation and releasing tension.

## Pressure Points In The Gua Sha Therapy Practice

Gua sha therapy focuses on specific pressure points in the body that are believed to be connected to various health conditions. These pressure points are usually along the meridians, or energy pathways, of the body. Pressing and scraping these areas with a stone or other tool can help to stimulate circulation and release tension. It is important to be aware of the sensitivity of the skin in these areas and to use light pressure when using Gua sha.

## The Benefits

The benefits of Gua sha therapy include improved circulation, reduced inflammation, increased energy levels, better sleep quality, improved mental clarity, and more. Additionally, it can be helpful in reducing chronic pain and soothing emotional stress. It is a safe and natural way to help improve overall health and well-being.

Gua sha therapy can be used on its own or in combination with other healing modalities, such as acupuncture, herbal medicine, massage, aromatherapy, and more. It is important to find a qualified practitioner who has been trained in the use of Gua sha tools and techniques.

## Reiki

Reiki and reflexology are both holistic healing modalities that can help to relax the body, reduce stress, and promote well-being. Reiki is an energy therapy in which a practitioner channels universal energy through their hands into the recipient's body. This helps to balance the body's energy centres or chakras, allowing for a greater sense of peace and relaxation. Reflexology is a massage technique that uses pressure points on the hands, feet, and ears to stimulate corresponding points on the body's energy pathways. This can help to reduce stress, improve circulation, relieve pain, increase relaxation, and promote overall health.

Both Reiki and reflexology can be used in combination to create a more powerful healing experience. When practiced together, the energy healing of Reiki can be used to open up and balance the body's energy pathways, while reflexology can be used to stimulate and activate them further. By combining these two modalities, practitioners can create an even deeper sense of relaxation for their clients or patients.

### Benefits Of Reiki

Reiki offers a multitude of benefits, enhancing overall well-being and promoting a balanced life. One of the key advantages of Reiki is stress reduction. The universal energy flowing through the body during a Reiki session can help to soothe anxiety and alleviate stress, cultivating a sense of deep relaxation. Additionally, Reiki can be instrumental in pain management. Numerous people report a reduction in pain and discomfort following a Reiki session, which can be particularly beneficial for those suffering from chronic pain conditions. Reiki also aids in improving sleep patterns, promoting better sleep quality and, consequently, a more energized waking state. Importantly, Reiki works in harmony with all other medical or therapeutic techniques and can assist in relieving side effects and promoting recovery. Thus, it can be a valuable addition to traditional medical treatments, providing emotional and physical support to the healing process.

**How Reiki Works**

Reiki is based on the idea that an unseen life force energy flows through all living things. This life force energy, also known as 'Ki', can be blocked by physical and emotional stressors or illness. In a Reiki session, practitioners send healing energy to restore equilibrium in the body by allowing Ki to flow freely again. Reiki is a non-invasive therapy, so there are no physical manipulations involved. It is simple and natural, allowing the body to heal itself when it's ready. While there is no scientific proof of Reiki's effectiveness, many people report feeling relaxed, more positive thoughts and an improved sense of well-being after a Reiki session.

## The Tools

Reiki practitioners use traditional symbols and techniques to assist them in their practice. The most common tools include hand positions, chanting, sacred mantras and prayer. Hand positions are placed on various parts of the body where energy is believed to be blocked or stagnant. This provides a sense of relaxation as the practitioner channels Ki from their hands to the recipient's body. Chanting, mantras and prayer is used to send positive energy and intention into the session.

## Pressure Points In Reiki

In Reiki, pressure points are used to target specific parts of the body. These points provide access to Ki energy and can be beneficial for calming the mind and promoting relaxation. Common pressure points include:

### Third Eye Point

Third Eye Point is often the first pressure point used in Reiki sessions. It helps to balance and focus energy, while allowing practitioners to connect with their intuition. This can be particularly beneficial for those seeking guidance or direction in their spiritual journey.

### Crown Point

The Crown Point is located at the top of the

head and can be a powerful point for relaxation. Stimulating this point helps to release tension in the body while promoting spiritual connection. It can also help to connect with inner wisdom, allowing practitioners and recipients to gain insight into their life's purpose.

## Solar Plexus Point

The Solar Plexus Point is located at the center of the abdomen and can be used to relieve stress and anxiety. Stimulating this point helps to promote feelings of confidence, empowerment, and inner strength. It also encourages an increase in self-esteem and clarity of thought.

## Heart Chakra Point

The Heart Chakra Point is located in the center of the chest and helps to promote feelings of love and compassion. Stimulating this point can help to open up the heart, allowing energy to flow freely, encouraging transformation and healing.

## Sacral Chakra Point

The Sacral Chakra Point is located just below the navel and can be used to stimulate creativity and intuition. Stimulating this point helps to balance emotional energy and can be beneficial for those dealing with blockages in creativity.

## Root Chakra Point

The Root Chakra Point is located at the base

of the spine and helps to ground energy in the body. Stimulating this point can give a sense of stability, while encouraging feelings of safety and protection.

Overall, Reiki and reflexology can be powerful tools for relaxation and healing. By combining these two modalities, practitioners can create a truly transformative experience for their clients or patients. Whether used as an alternative therapy or in combination with traditional medical treatments, Reiki can help to reduce stress, improve circulation, reduce pain, increase relaxation, and promote overall health.

**Vertical Reflex Therapy**

Vertical Reflex Therapy (VRT) is a powerful form of reflexology that is based on the principle that the feet and hands are connected to different parts of the body, allowing for gentle yet effective natural healing. It works by massaging and stimulating the reflex points on the feet which correspond to particular organs in order to improve both physical and emotional well-being. This massage works on a deeper level to stimulate the natural healing process in the body, restoring balance and providing relief from various conditions. VRT is suitable for people of all ages and can be used to treat a variety of issues such as arthritis, chronic fatigue syndrome, digestive problems, depression and many others.

## Benefits Of Vertical Reflex Therapy

The benefits of Vertical Reflex Therapy are numerous. One of the key benefits is that it can provide natural pain relief from a wide range of conditions such as fibromyalgia, arthritis, and back pain. Additionally, VRT helps to stimulate circulation and reduce tension in muscles. This can help improve sleep quality and provide better overall health for those suffering from insomnia or anxiety.

VRT is also known for being a safe and non-invasive therapy. It is easy to learn, relatively inexpensive, and can be self-administered from the comfort of your own home. Furthermore, VRT does not involve any drugs or surgery, making it an attractive option for those looking for natural pain relief solutions.

VRT can also help improve posture and balance as well as increase flexibility and mobility. Through this therapy, individuals are able to improve their overall physical and mental well-being. This can in turn have a positive effect on energy levels, performance, and mood.

## The Reflex Meridian Therapy

Reflex Meridian Therapy is a form of massage that focuses on the meridians and reflex points of the body. It works by stimulating these points to help restore balance in the body and promote healing.

The therapist uses their hands to apply pressure to specific areas of the body, oftentimes using reflexology tools like balls or other objects. This helps to open up energy pathways, reduce tension, and alleviate pain. The therapist may also use heat or cold to enhance the effects of the massage.

The theory behind Reflex Meridian Therapy is that it helps to balance the body's qi (or 'chi') energy flow. By restoring balance in the body's energy pathways, it helps to promote both physical and mental well-being.

The benefits of Reflex Meridian Therapy vary from person to person, but some of the most common include:

**Improved Circulation**

Reflex Meridian Therapy helps to improve circulation by stimulating the nerve endings that are located in the feet and hands. As these nerves become activated, they promote better blood flow throughout the body, which can provide relief from soreness or pain. This improved circulation can also deliver increased levels of energy to the body's cells, helping them to function more efficiently and providing an overall feeling of well-being.

Improved sleep quality

Stimulating the reflex points helps to reduce tension and anxiety, which can improve sleep quality. It is also believed that Reflex Meridian Therapy helps to regulate hormones, which can help to promote better restful sleep.

### Reduced Pain And Inflammation In Muscles And Joints

The massage techniques used in Reflex Meridian Therapy can help to reduce muscular tension, aches and pains. It also helps to improve the range of motion in joints and muscles, which can provide relief from stiffness and soreness.

### Reduction Of Headaches Or Migraines

Massaging the reflex points can help to reduce stress and tension in the body, which is a major cause of headaches or migraines. As such, Reflex Meridian Therapy can help to relieve headache symptoms and reduce the frequency of migraine attacks.

### Improved Digestion

Reflexology massage stimulates nerve endings in the digestive system, which helps to improve digestion and absorption of nutrients from food. This improved digestive process helps to regulate bowel movements as well as prevent constipation and bloating.

### Reduced Fatigue

Reflex Meridian Therapy helps to improve circulation, which can assist in reducing fatigue and promoting higher levels of energy throughout the day. It can also help to reduce stress levels, which is a major cause of fatigue.

Overall, Reflex Meridian Therapy can be beneficial for anyone looking to promote general well-being. It is not intended to diagnose or treat any medical condition, but can help to reduce pain and improve overall health and wellbeing.

It is important to consult with your healthcare provider before beginning any form of massage therapy, as it can be contraindicated in some conditions. It is also essential to be sure that the therapist you choose has the proper qualifications and experience to provide Reflex Meridian Therapy safely and effectively.

By taking advantage of the many benefits of Reflex Meridian Therapy, you can help to promote overall health and well-being. With the right therapist, you can enjoy improved quality of life and a more balanced body and mind.

### The Morell Technique Of Reflexology

The Morell Technique is a method of reflexology based on the idea that all parts of the body are interconnected. It seeks to rebalance the flow of energy in the body by stimulating points located around the feet, hands, and ears. By doing so, it aims to improve overall health and well-being through reducing stress and tension, relieving pain, and stimulating the body's healing process.

This technique works by applying pressure to the feet in specific areas. Reflexology charts can be used to identify where these points are located on each foot. When the practitioner applies pressure to a certain point, it is believed that this stimulates energy flow throughout the body. The practitioner may use their hands, fingers, or a special reflexology device to apply pressure.

The practitioner can also use the Morell Technique on the hands and ears. Different points of each body part are said to correspond with certain organs and areas of the body, which practitioners must knowers know where these points are located in order for them to be effective.

This technique has been used to treat a wide range of ailments, from chronic pain to nausea and digestive issues. While it is not backed by any scientific evidence, many people believe that this type of reflexology can provide relief. If you are interested in trying the Morell Technique for yourself, make sure to find an experienced practitioner who has been trained in the technique.

**Benefits Of Morell Technique Of Reflexology Include:**

- Relief of pain and other ailments
- Reduces stress and tension in the body
- Improves overall wellbeing

- Stimulates healing process
- Can be used to treat a variety of issues, including digestive problems, headaches, nausea, and more.

The Morell Technique is an ancient form of reflexology that has been used for centuries to treat various conditions. While it is important to note that there is no scientific evidence to back up the claims of reflexology, many people believe that this type of alternative medicine can be effective in treating a variety of ailments. If you are interested in trying the Morell Technique for yourself, make sure to find an experienced practitioner who has been trained in the technique.

**Crystal Healing**

Crystal healing is an ancient practice that involves using crystals to improve physical, mental, emotional and spiritual wellness. It is believed that the energy of a crystal can be absorbed through the skin in order to affect a person's health. Reflexology is a form of massage therapy that uses precise pressure points on the feet, hands and ears to promote relaxation and healing. It is believed that these pressure points are connected to different parts of the body, allowing for improved circulation and relief from pain.

When used together, crystal healing and reflexology can be a powerful combination for promoting good health. The energy of crystals amplifies the effects of massage therapy, while the massage itself helps to improve circulation in areas that may have become blocked due to stress or trauma. This allows for more efficient exchange of energy between the body and the crystals, creating a positive healing effect on physical, mental and emotional levels.

In addition to providing relaxation and relief from pain, combining crystal healing with reflexology can also help to balance out energies in the body. This helps to bring harmony into all areas of life, including relationships, career and overall well-being.

Crystal healing and reflexology can be used to treat a variety of conditions such as chronic pain, stress, insomnia, anxiety and depression. It is important to select the right crystals for each individual person in order to get the most out of this type of therapy. A qualified crystal healer or reflexologist will be able to advise the best type of crystals and techniques for each individual.

Crystal healing and reflexology can provide a powerful way to improve physical, mental, emotional and spiritual health. By combining these two ancient practices together, it is possible to create a unique healing experience that can be tailored to meet your individual needs.

**How Crystal Healing Works**

Crystal healing works by harnessing the energy

of crystals to restore balance in the body. Every crystal has its own unique frequency and vibration that can be used to influence different areas of life. By placing crystals on or near the body, these vibrations can be absorbed into the cells and organs, allowing for improved circulation and a sense of relaxation.

When combined with massage therapy, the effects of crystal healing are amplified. The massage helps to work out any blockages in the body, while the energy of the crystals amplifies this effect. This creates a powerful combination that can help to heal physical, mental and emotional issues.

It is important to use the correct type of crystals for each individual person in order to ensure that the effects are beneficial. A qualified crystal healer or reflexologist will be able to advise the best type of crystals and techniques for each individual.

### Sound Therapy Through Reflexology

Reflexology is an ancient practice that has been used to promote healing and relaxation for thousands of years. It is based on the belief that each part of the body is connected with points or "reflexes" in the hands, feet, and ears. By applying pressure to these reflex points, it is believed that a person can improve their physical and emotional health, as well as alleviate pain.

Sound therapy is a modern form of reflexology that uses sound waves to stimulate the body's natural healing processes. It works by sending sound vibrations through the body which are said to balance the energy centers of the body and help to promote harmony and wellbeing. In addition to helping with common ailments like headaches, sound therapy can also help to reduce stress and anxiety.

To experience the benefits of sound therapy through reflexology, practitioners will use special tools such as tuning forks or singing bowls to send vibrations into the body. They may also incorporate other techniques such as massage, yoga, or meditation into the practice.

The effects of sound therapy on physical and emotional well-being are still being investigated, but some studies have suggested that it can be beneficial for people suffering from chronic pain or stress-related conditions. Additionally, sound therapy may help to increase levels of relaxation and improve overall quality of life.

**How Sound Therapy Works**

Sound therapy works by introducing vibrations into the body and using those vibrations to create a harmonious balance within. By sending sound waves through specific areas, practitioners can help to promote relaxation, reduce inflammation, and stimulate healing. The intensity of the vibration will depend on the type of instrument used, as well as the practitioner's skill level.

In addition to using instruments, practitioners may incorporate other techniques such as visualization or guided meditation into sound therapy. Visualization involves creating an image in your mind of a calming place or situation while guided meditation helps to focus the mind on positive thoughts and ideas.

**Ear Candling**

It is no surprise that ear candling and reflexology go hand-in-hand. Ear candling is an ancient practice, believed to help remove toxins from the body as well as improve overall health. By placing a lit candle in the ear canal, it creates a vacuum effect that can draw out impurities from within the ear.

Reflexology can help aid in the process of ear candling. When applying pressure to specific areas of the foot that correspond to the ears, it can help unblock and cleanse any toxins from around the ear and reduce pain. This is further enhanced when combined with other therapeutic treatments such as acupressure or massage.

In addition to its cleansing properties, ear candling can also be used to treat ear infections, sinus infections and other health concerns. It is important to note that ear candling should only be done by a qualified professional who has experience in the practice. It is not recommended to perform this treatment without consulting with a specialist first.

Ear candling combined with reflexology can help bring balance to the body and improve overall well-being. It is important to remember that it should only be done under the supervision of a qualified professional to ensure safety and maximum benefit.

At the end of the procedure, it is recommended to use ear drops or oil on your ears in order to help lubricate them after being treated with ear candling. This will also help to prevent any further infections or pain.

Reflexology can help bring balance and harmony to the body, while ear candling can help cleanse and detoxify it. Together they are an effective way of treating various ailments and restoring health. It is important to remember that both disciplines should be done under the supervision of a qualified professional for maximum benefit.

**The Tools**

In order to properly and safely perform ear candling, it is important to have the right supplies and tools. This includes candles specifically designed for this purpose, as well as oil or drops to lubricate the ears after the treatment. Additionally, cotton swabs may be needed in order to clean up any debris that may come out during the procedure.

## Pressure Points In Ear Candling

When performing ear candling with reflexology, it is important to be aware of the pressure points that are associated with each. In particular, there are three main pressure points in the ears that correspond to reflexology: the Erb's point, which controls the movement of energy and blood circulation; Shen Men, which helps to open up blocked channels; and the Triple Warmer point, which helps to regulate heat and energy in the body.

By pressing down on these pressure points during ear candling, it can help increase the effectiveness of both treatments. Additionally, this can help to reduce pain and discomfort from the ear canal area as well.

It is important to note that when performing ear candling with reflexology, it is best to do so in a comfortable and relaxing environment. This will help ensure that the treatments are effective and beneficial, while also reducing any discomfort or stress. Additionally, it is important to remember to listen to your body when performing these treatments - if something does not feel right, then stop immediately.

# CHAPTER 8: OTHER TECHNIQUES USED IN REFLEXOLOGY

Basic hand and finger movements

When it comes to practicing basic movements in reflexology, the hands and fingers are key. The most common hand and finger techniques used in reflexology include thumb walking, hooking, stretching and rotating.

Thumb walking is a technique where the practitioner uses their thumbs on pressure points of areas of the body that require healing or relief from pain. The thumb is used to apply a small amount of pressure to the area and then moved in a circular motion along the body part.

Hooking is another commonly used technique in reflexology, which involves using the index finger and thumb to hook onto an area of the body. Hooking can be used for stimulating various areas or can be used as a form of massage therapy.

Stretching is another common technique in reflexology which involves using the index finger and thumb to stretch various areas on the body. This technique is used to promote circulation and can be used to help reduce muscle tension and stiffness.

Rotating is a technique that combines stretching

with thumb walking. It involves using the thumbs to rotate in a circular motion over different parts of the body. This technique is great for promoting relaxation and can be used to increase circulation.

## Thumb Walking

Thumb walking is a type of reflexology technique used to provide relief from tension and pain in the different parts of the hand. It involves applying gentle pressure with the thumb along specific pressure points, stimulating nerve endings and providing relief to various aches and pains. Thumb walking is an effective way to relax tense muscles, improve circulation, reduce stress levels, and help the body heal itself. It can also be used to provide relief from pain and inflammation in the hands, wrists, and fingers.

## Steps Of Thumb Walking

When performing thumb walking, it's important to begin in the same place each time in order to achieve consistent results. The steps for thumb walking are as follows:

1) Start by applying gentle pressure with your thumb along the base of the palm and move up towards the fingertips. Make sure you keep a steady rhythm throughout this movement.

2) Focus on each finger individually, starting with the thumb and working your way up to the pinky.

3) Massage each individual finger from base to

tip, including the joints as well as any areas that feel tight or sore. You can also gently press the fingernails in order to stimulate nerve endings and provide further relief.

4) When you are done working on each finger, move back to the base of the palm and massage in circular motions. Be careful not to press too hard as this can cause discomfort.

5) Finally, finish by giving each hand a light massage using your fingertips. This will help relax any tension that has built up during the procedure and promote further healing.

**Hooking**

Hooking is a technique used in reflexology that involves using the index finger and thumb to hook onto an area of the body. It can be used for stimulating different areas or as a form of massage therapy. This technique is great for relieving tension, increasing circulation, and improving flexibility.

When performing hooking, it's important to use light pressure and to always keep the thumb and index finger hooked together. The movements should be slow and steady, with the practitioner focusing on each area of the body for around 30 seconds before moving onto another area.

**Steps Of Hooking**

Hooking can be used on parts of the body such

as the neck, shoulders, back, and legs. To perform hooking correctly, follow these steps:

1) Using your index finger and thumb, gently hook onto the area you wish to massage.

2) Gently move your hands in a circular motion for around 30 seconds.

3) Repeat this motion on different areas of the body, focusing on each area for around 30 seconds before moving onto another one.

4) When you are finished with the massage, gently rub the area to help relax any remaining tension and to improve circulation.

## Stretching

Stretching is a type of reflexology technique used to promote circulation and reduce muscle tension and stiffness. It involves using the index finger and thumb to stretch various areas of the body. This technique is great for improving flexibility, relieving pain, increasing range of motion, and helping the body heal itself.

When performing stretching techniques in reflexology, it's important to use a light touch in order to avoid excessive pressure. The movements should be slow and steady in order to achieve the best results.

## Steps Of Stretching

When performing stretching, it's important to

focus on each area for at least 30 seconds before moving onto another one. To properly stretch an area, follow these steps:

1) Using your index finger and thumb, gently stretch the area you wish to massage.

2) Gently move your hands in a circular motion for around 30 seconds.

3) Repeat this motion on different areas of the body, focusing on each area for around 30 seconds before moving onto another one.

4) When you are finished with the massage, gently rub the area to help relax any remaining tension and to improve circulation.

**Rotating**

Rotating is a technique used in reflexology that combines stretching with thumb walking. It involves using the thumbs to rotate in a circular motion over different parts of the body. This technique is great for promoting relaxation and can be used to increase circulation.

When performing rotating techniques in reflexology, it's important to use a light touch in order to avoid excessive pressure. The movements should be slow and steady in order to achieve the best results.

steps of Rotating

When performing rotating techniques, it's

important to focus on each area for at least 30 seconds before moving onto another one. To properly rotate an area, follow these steps:

1) Using your thumbs, gently rotate the area you wish to massage.

2) Gently move your hands in a circular motion for around 30 seconds.

3) Repeat this motion on different areas of the body, focusing on each area for around 30 seconds before moving onto another one.

4) When you are finished with the massage, gently rub the area to help relax any remaining tension and to improve circulation.

## Specific Pressure Points And Areas On The Feet, Hands, And Ears

Reflexology is an ancient practice that works on the principle of applying pressure to certain areas of the feet, hands and ears. Through these techniques, practitioners seek to provide relief from a variety of ailments. It has been used for centuries as part of traditional Chinese medicine and some modern treatments such as massage therapy.

The main goal of reflexology is to access points on the body that are believed to be linked to organs, systems and energy pathways. By working on these points, practitioners are able to relax the individual and promote healing.

The reflexologist will use their hands to locate pressure points in various parts of the body. For example, on the feet they may press certain areas such as the toes, heel or arch; on the hands, they may press areas such as the palm, fingers or knuckles; and on the ears, they may press certain points.

The specific pressure points and techniques used in reflexology vary depending on the practitioner. Generally, though, practitioners will use a light touch to stimulate various points on the body in order to provide relief from pain or tension.

It is important to note that reflexology is not a stand-alone treatment and should be used in conjunction with other medical treatments. It can, however, provide some relief from stress, tension or pain when used regularly.

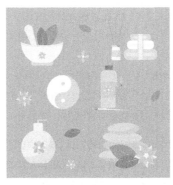

**The Sequence Of Application For Optimal Results**

Sequence of application for optimal results is an extremely important component of reflexology and should be taken into account when performing the practice. When done properly, the sequence can maximize the benefits of reflexology, allowing for quicker and more effective results.

In order to get the best outcome from Reflexology, it is important to follow a few simple steps:

1. Begin by applying light pressure with your hands and/or fingers to the specific reflex points.
2. Perform circular massage movements with your thumb or finger in a clockwise direction, using slow, gentle motions that flow from one point to another.
3. Pause for several minutes at each pressure point before proceeding to the next one. This will allow time for the body's energy pathways to activate and open up.
4. Use the correct pressure when applying reflexology, using your discretion as to how much pressure is necessary for each individual point.
5. Work through all of the reflex points in sequence until the session has been completed.
6. When finished, allow yourself to relax and become aware of any changes that may have occurred during the session.

Reflexology is a safe and effective way to promote health, well-being and relaxation. By following the correct sequence of applications for optimal results, you can experience its many benefits.

# CHAPTER 9: BABY REFLEX

B aby Reflex
Baby Reflex is a form of reflexology specifically used to promote better health and overall well-being in infants. This practice uses gentle massage techniques to stimulate specific points on the baby's feet, hands, and head that are believed to correspond with different parts of the body, such as organs or glands. Practised professionally by trained and certified reflexologists, Baby Reflex is a safe and natural way to provide relief from pain or discomfort, help improve digestion and circulation, strengthen the immune system, and promote better sleep.

## Benefits Of Baby Reflex

### Improved digestive health
Baby Reflex is a great way to take care of the digestive health of your baby. By stimulating specific points on the hands and feet that are related to the stomach, Baby Reflex can help reduce colic and other digestive problems. This gentle massage techniques may also help improve digestion by increasing blood flow in the abdominal area which can lead to an increase in absorption of nutrients from the food. In addition, Baby Reflex can help reduce constipation and

bloating by helping to relax the muscles in the digestive tract.

## Reduced Stress

A reflexology session for your baby can also be a great way to reduce stress. The gentle massage techniques used during a reflexology session can provide instant calming effects that help relieve tension and anxiety in babies. This can help them feel more relaxed and content, which can contribute to better sleep and improved overall well-being.

## Better Circulation

Gently massaging the feet and hands of your baby during a reflexology session can also help improve their circulation. By increasing blood flow throughout the body, this could lead to improved concentration and motor skills as well as a strengthened immune system.

## Improved Immunity

Stimulating certain reflex points on the feet and head can help strengthen the baby's immune system, allowing them to better fight off illnesses. This can help them stay healthier and more energetic, which is essential for their growth and development.

## Better Sleep

Babies who receive Baby Reflex often experience

improved quality of sleep due to the relaxation effects of massage and reflexology. This can help them get the rest they need for optimal growth and development, which is essential for their overall health and well-being.

**For Teething :**

Massaging the feet and hands can help soothe sore gums and reduce discomfort. Additionally, reflexology can improve digestion and circulation in teething babies, which can help them feel more comfortable and relaxed. It's important to practice gentle massage on the areas associated with teething such as the toes, heels, and fingertips. If your baby is uncomfortable with the massage, it's best to stop and try again at another time.

**For Whole-Body Benefit :**

Baby Reflex is an excellent way to provide whole-body benefits for your baby. The gentle massage techniques used during a reflexology session can help reduce stress, improve circulation and digestion, strengthen the immune system, and promote better sleep. With regular practice, these beneficial effects will accumulate over time and can contribute to a healthier lifestyle for your child.

**For Parents :**

In addition to the numerous benefits for your baby, Baby Reflex can also be a great way for parents to bond with their child. The calming and soothing effects of massage will create a special moment between you and your baby that can help strengthen the bond between you. It's also an excellent opportunity to connect with nature and promote better health through natural means.

## How Does It Work?

Baby Reflex works by stimulating specific points on the baby's feet, hands, and head that are believed to correspond with different parts of the body. A reflexology practitioner will use gentle massage techniques on these points to promote better circulation and relaxation. By increasing blood flow to specific areas, this can help improve digestion, reduce stress, strengthen the immune system, and provide relief from pain or discomfort.

## Tips For Getting Started

When getting started with Baby Reflex, it's important to find a certified and experienced reflexologist who specializes in baby reflexology. This will ensure that your baby is receiving the best possible care. It's also important to talk to your doctor about any potential risks or contraindications before beginning treatment. Additionally, it's a good idea to create an environment that is conducive to relaxation, such as playing calming music or providing a comfortable space for your baby.

## When To Start Baby Reflexology?

You can start introducing reflexology to your baby as early as the first few weeks of life. However, it's essential to ensure that the sessions are gentle and short. As your baby grows older and becomes more accustomed to the touch, these sessions can gradually become longer. It's always recommended to consult with a pediatrician before starting reflexology or any new health practices with your baby. Remember, every baby is unique, and what works for one may not necessarily work for another. Therefore, it's important to observe your child's reaction during and after the session to ensure the experience is positive and beneficial.

### Safety Considerations

Baby Reflex should only be practiced by a certified and experienced reflexologist who specializes in baby reflexology. It's also important to familiarize yourself with the safety guidelines for performing reflexology on babies before beginning treatment.

It's essential to ensure that the sessions are gentle and short, as too much pressure or stimulation may lead to discomfort or even pain in some cases. Additionally, it's important to observe your child's reaction during and after the session to ensure the experience is positive and beneficial. It's recommended to stop the session if your baby becomes fussy or agitated, as this could indicate that they are not comfortable with the treatment.

Overall, Baby Reflex can be a great way to take care of your baby's health and well-being. With the right approach, it can provide numerous benefits that can contribute to their overall growth and development. If you have any questions or concerns about Baby Reflex, make sure to talk to your doctor before trying this method of treatment.

## Specific Pressure Points And Areas On The Feet, Hands, And Ears

### Head

Head reflexology focuses on areas of the head that correspond to other parts of the body. These points are typically located on top of the head, near the temples, and behind the ears. Pressure points in these areas can help alleviate stress and tension as well as improve digestion, circulation, and immunity.

### Temples

The temples are key points in head reflexology that can be used to relieve headaches, stress, and fatigue. Stimulating these specific areas on the side of the head with gentle massage techniques can help promote relaxation and better energy levels.

## Forehead

The forehead is another area of the head that can be used in reflexology to help reduce stress, tension, and headaches. Applying gentle pressure on these points can help improve circulation and increase alertness.

## Crown Of The Head

The crown of the head is a key point in head reflexology that can help improve overall health and well-being. Stimulating this area with massage techniques can help reduce stress, promote better sleep, and strengthen the immune system.

## The Base Of The Skull

The base of the skull is another important area for head reflexology. Applying gentle massage on this specific point can help reduce tension and fatigue as well as soothe headaches and discomfort.

## Feet

The feet are the primary focus for reflexology, as they contain numerous pressure points that correspond to different areas of the body. By stimulating these points with gentle massage techniques, it can help improve circulation and reduce stress and tension.

## Big Toe

The big toe is an important point in foot reflexology that corresponds to the head. Stimulating this area with massage techniques can help reduce headaches and tension as well as improve alertness, clarity, and concentration.

## Ball Of The Foot

The ball of the foot is another important point in reflexology that corresponds to the digestive system. Massaging this area can help with digestion and appetite as well as promote better sleep.

## Heel

The heel is a key point in foot reflexology that corresponds to the lower back. Stimulating this area with massage techniques can help reduce lower back pain and discomfort as well as promote better circulation.

## Ankles

The ankles are another important area for foot reflexology that can be used to treat various conditions, including headaches, insomnia, and digestive issues. Applying pressure to the ankles can help reduce stress and tension as well as improve circulation and immunity.

## Hands

The hands are also important points in reflexology that correspond to different areas of the body.

Stimulating these specific areas with massage techniques can help promote relaxation, reduce stress, and improve circulation.

**Thumb**

The thumb is the primary point in hand reflexology that corresponds to the head. Applying pressure to this specific area can help reduce headaches and tension as well as improve concentration and alertness.

**Fingers**

The fingers are another important area for hand reflexology that can be used to treat a variety of conditions. Stimulating these points with massage techniques can help with digestion, sleep, and stress-related disorders.

**Palm**

The palm of the hand is a key point in reflexology that corresponds to the heart. Massaging this area can help reduce stress and tension as well as improve circulation and blood pressure.

**Wrists**

The wrists are another important point in hand reflexology that can be used to treat a variety of conditions. Stimulating these points with massage techniques can help reduce stress and tension, as well as improve circulation throughout the body.

## Ears

The ears are also important points in reflexology that correspond to different areas of the body. Applying gentle pressure on specific areas of the ear can help promote relaxation, reduce stress and tension, and improve overall health and well-being.

## Lobe

The lobe is a key point in ear reflexology that corresponds to the reproductive system. Massaging this area can help with fertility issues, menstrual cramps, and hormonal imbalances.

## Tragus

The tragus is another important point in ear reflexology that corresponds to the digestive system. Stimulating this area with massage techniques can help improve digestion and appetite as well as reduce stress and tension.

## Helix

The helix is a key point in ear reflexology that corresponds to the immune system. Applying gentle pressure on this specific area can help strengthen the immune system, alleviate stress, and improve overall health.

Baby Reflexology can be a great way to promote overall well-being in your little one. Stimulating the reflex points on their feet, hands, and ears with gentle massage techniques can help reduce tension and fatigue as well as boost immunity and circulation—all of which are essential for their growth and development.

# CHAPTER 10: WHO SHOULD NOT HAVE REFLEXOLOGY?

Reflexology is not recommended for everyone because it may not be safe in certain cases. Generally, reflexology should be avoided if you:

## Have Any Kind Of Infection Or Injury On Your Feet

Having an infection or injury on your feet does not make it advisable to get reflexology. The therapist applies pressure to specific areas on the feet, which may aggravate any existing foot infections or injuries. Moreover, an open wound could potentially become a route for further infections, making the situation worse. It is essential to allow your feet to heal completely before seeking reflexology treatment. Always consult with a healthcare provider before starting any new treatment.

## Are Pregnant Or Have Had A Recent Surgery

Due to the potentially high levels of pressure used in reflexology, it is not recommended for anyone who is pregnant or has recently undergone any kind of surgery. The increased pressure may be too uncomfortable for individuals with such conditions. Moreover, certain areas of the feet can cause contractions, which is why some therapists choose not to work on pregnant clients.

### Take Blood Thinners Like Aspirin, Ibuprofen, Warfarin, And Others

Individuals taking medications that thin the blood are advised to refrain from reflexology since it could potentially cause excessive bleeding and bruising due to the pressure applied during a session. If you take any medications that thin the blood, consult with your doctor before trying reflexology.

### Have Certain Medical Conditions Such As Diabetes, Cancer, Heart Disease, Or High Blood Pressure

Individuals suffering from specific diseases and chronic conditions are advised to avoid reflexology since it could potentially aggravate these ailments. As an example, those with diabetes should not receive reflexology as it could potentially interfere with their blood sugar levels. Similarly, those with high blood pressure may find the treatment too stimulating and should therefore avoid reflexology sessions.

### Have A History Of Joint Problems Like Rheumatoid Arthritis

If you suffer from a condition such as rheumatoid arthritis, then reflexology may not be suitable for you. The pressure used in a reflexology session can be too much for those with joint problems, and may therefore aggravate the ailment. It is advisable to speak to your doctor before trying reflexology if you have any kind of joint problem.

It is important to note that even if none of the above applies to you, there are still certain instances where reflexology may not be suitable for you. Therefore, it is always best to consult with a healthcare provider before starting any treatment. This will help ensure that you receive the best possible care and attention for your particular needs.

**Thyroid Problems**

While reflexology is generally considered safe for most individuals, those with certain thyroid problems should exercise caution. Overstimulation of the reflex points corresponding to the thyroid gland may potentially alter hormone levels or exacerbate existing conditions. Therefore, it is of paramount importance that individuals with thyroid issues consult their healthcare provider before engaging in reflexology treatment.

**Epilepsy**

Similarly, reflexology should also be avoided by people with epilepsy due to the potential for seizure activity. Stimulation of the reflex points corresponding to the nervous system may aggravate epileptic seizures. It is recommended that individuals diagnosed with epilepsy talk to their doctor prior to beginning a reflexology session.

**A Low Platelet Count Or Other Blood Disorders**

For individuals with a low platelet count or other blood disorders, the effects of reflexology on the circulatory system may be dangerous. Reflexology is known to increase circulation in the body and thus can make some pre-existing conditions worse. Accordingly, people with existing blood disorders should err on the side of caution and consult their healthcare provider before receiving reflexology treatments.

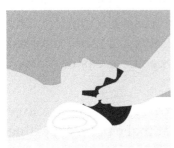

**Massage Vs. Reflexology: What's The Difference?**

When it comes to massage and reflexology, many people are unsure of what the differences between them are. Massage therapy is used to ease physical pain through the manipulation of soft body tissues such as muscles and connective tissue. It can help reduce stress, improve relaxation and circulation, as well as help create a feeling of balance in the body. Reflexology works on the same principle but instead concentrates on specific points within the feet, hands and ears that have corresponding areas in other parts of the body.

Reflexology is a more targeted approach than massage therapy, as it focuses exclusively on points that are believed to correspond with certain organs and bodily structures. The therapist applies pressure to these areas, which then causes a reaction elsewhere in the body. This can be used to treat pain, reduce stress, and improve overall health.

The main difference between massage therapy and reflexology is that massage therapy works on the entire body while reflexology focuses on specific points within the body. Massage therapy can help to reduce inflammation, improve flexibility and range of motion, increase circulation, and promote relaxation. Reflexology is more targeted and can be used to treat specific areas of pain or discomfort.

Ultimately, both massage therapy and reflexology have their own benefits that make them appealing for different reasons. Depending on your individual needs, either one could be the right choice for you. Talk to your doctor or a certified reflexologist to discuss which approach would be best suited to your needs, and make sure that any practitioner you visit is qualified and licensed in their field.

**What You Can Expect During A Reflexology**

## Session ?

As a reflexologist, your therapist will use their hands to apply pressure to different areas of your feet and hands. They may also use various instruments such as massage rollers or wooden sticks. During the session, the therapist will ask questions about your health history and any issues you are having in order to determine which areas of the feet require special attention.

The session usually lasts for about an hour. During this time, your therapist will focus on specific areas of the feet that are associated with different organs and systems in the body. For example, they may focus on pressure points related to digestion or circulation issues.

Your reflexologist will provide a detailed explanation of what is happening during the session and how it may help relieve stress and bring relaxation. They will also explain what areas of the feet to focus on in order to bring balance back into the body.

At the end of the session, your therapist will offer advice on lifestyle changes that can be made in order to maintain physical and mental well-being. This may include changes such as diet, exercise, or even homoeopathy.

### How Long Before You Start Seeing Benefits?

In general, reflexology is thought to be a

relatively quick-acting form of treatment—many people report feeling better after just one session. However, some individuals may require multiple sessions before they begin to feel any positive effects.

One way to gauge whether or not reflexology is working is to keep track of your symptoms before and during the course of treatment. For instance, if you're experiencing stress-related headaches, note the number or frequency of headaches before starting reflexology, and then compare that to how often they occur after a few sessions. If you feel that your symptoms are improving with each session, reflexology is likely to have a beneficial effect.

Another approach to measuring the effectiveness of reflexology is to keep a journal and track how you feel after each session. Note any changes in your physical or mental state, and if you can identify patterns that correlate with the sessions, then it's likely that reflexology is helping you.

Ultimately, whether or not reflexology is working depends on your individual needs and circumstances. Keeping track of your symptoms before, during, and after treatment can help you to determine whether or not you're experiencing the benefits of reflexology.

# CHAPTER 11: PERFORMERS

Reflexology practitioners, often referred to as reflexologists, may be licensed in many states and can include massage therapists and chiropractors. In some cases, a reflexologist's license can be included with one of these other disciplines. Reflexology practitioners typically focus on the feet while performing this technique, although they may also work on hands or ears. Practitioners may use a variety of techniques, such as applying pressure to certain points on the body, using specific massage techniques or even incorporating aromatherapy into their practice. The goal of reflexology is to help restore balance within the body and bring relief from pain or discomfort.

The effectiveness of reflexology has been studied extensively and there is evidence that it can be beneficial for conditions such as headaches, stress, digestive issues and joint pain. In addition to providing relief from physical symptoms, reflexology may also help to improve a person's overall well-being. This holistic approach provides both physical and emotional benefits that can be enjoyed long after the session has ended.

**Practitioners**

Reflexology practitioners use various techniques to apply pressure to the feet, hands, and

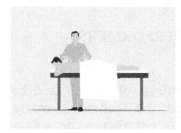

ears. These techniques vary from person to person and can range from gentle massages to deep-tissue manipulation. Reflexologists are trained in both traditional methods and modern approaches such as neuromuscular therapy. They may also incorporate other modalities such as aromatherapy and homeopathic remedies to create a holistic approach to healing the body.

While reflexology is not meant to replace medical care, it can be used as part of an overall health regimen. Practitioners often find that clients experience relief from a variety of conditions such as headaches, fatigue, lower back pain, and digestive issues after just one session. It has also been known to reduce stress levels and improve overall well-being.

In addition to regular sessions, reflexologists often provide educational materials about the art of reflexology. These may include instructional videos, articles, and books that teach clients how to use massage techniques at home. They can also provide tips on lifestyle changes that could help with certain conditions. By empowering their patients with knowledge and self-care tools, reflexologists allow them to take control of their own health.

## Who Are Acupuncturists?

Acupuncturists are healthcare professionals who specialize in using techniques such as acupuncture and reflexology to promote wellness and healing. Acupuncture is an ancient Chinese practice that involves the insertion of extremely thin needles into specific points on the body, to stimulate energy flow through and around areas known as meridians to correct imbalances in the body. Acupuncturists use traditional Chinese medicine and therapies to help alleviate pain, treat disease, and improve overall health.

## What Is The Role Of Acupuncturists?

Acupuncturists play an essential role in the health and well-being of their clients. In addition to providing therapeutic treatments, they may also provide lifestyle advice, education on nutrition and exercise, and referrals for further treatment if needed. Acupuncturists are trained to recognize signs of medical distress, such as elevated blood pressure levels or an irregular heartbeat. They are also well-versed in the use of herbs and natural remedies to help promote healing.

### Naturopathic Physicians

Naturopathic physicians are medical professionals who combine traditional healing methods with modern scientific medical knowledge. They emphasize the body's inherent ability to restore and maintain its own health. The practice of naturopathy can involve a broad range of treatments including herbal medicine, nutrition, hydrotherapy, homoeopathy, and reflexology. The latter is an intriguing element of naturopathic medicine as it focuses on manipulating specific reflex points on the foot to induce healing responses in corresponding parts of the body.

## What Is The Role Of Naturopathic Physicians?

Naturopathic physicians are responsible for diagnosing and treating a variety of medical conditions through the use of natural therapies. They employ various methods, depending on the health concern being addressed. Naturopathic approaches can involve dietary changes, lifestyle modifications, herbal medicine, homoeopathy, physical manipulation (e.g., massage and reflexology), hydrotherapy, and other alternative therapies. In addition, they may also provide education and counselling to patients in order to prevent the onset of future medical issues. As primary care practitioners, naturopathic physicians can also refer their patients to specialists when necessary. Ultimately, naturopathic physicians aim to restore balance within the body by promoting healthy living habits and natural healing methods.

In terms of reflexology, naturopathic physicians rely on the use of finger and thumb pressure to manipulate specific points on the feet. This technique is used to stimulate energy pathways that are connected to different parts of the body in order to promote health and healing. By manipulating these points, practitioners can help to restore balance within the body and address a variety of symptoms such as pain, inflammation, and tension.

## Chiropractors

Chiropractors are professionals who specialize in treating musculoskeletal conditions such as back pain, neck pain, headaches, and other ailments related to the spine. They may also be involved in sports medicine or physical therapy. Chiropractors often use a combination of manual manipulation, soft tissue techniques, stretching exercises, ergonomic advice, and lifestyle counselling to help their patients achieve optimum health. In addition, chiropractors may use other modalities such as ultrasound, electrical stimulation, laser therapy, and nutrition counselling to treat a variety of conditions. They are also trained in the diagnosis and management of certain orthopaedic disorders.

Chiropractors generally believe that the body is able to heal itself with proper alignment and manipulation of the joints. Thus, they focus on restoring balance and normal function of the body through spinal adjustments, soft tissue massage therapy, lifestyle changes, and other therapies. Chiropractors may also recommend lifestyle modifications and nutritional supplements to promote overall well-being.

Chiropractic treatment has been shown to be effective in relieving pain, improving range of motion, and reducing inflammation. It can also help improve posture and balance as well as strengthen the muscles and ligaments that support the spine. The effects are usually long-lasting, and many patients find that regular chiropractic care helps them maintain good health.

Ultimately, chiropractors focus on restoring normal body function and promoting overall health and wellness. By helping patients achieve optimal alignment of the spine, chiropractic treatment can help reduce pain, improve range of motion, prevent injury, and promote accelerated healing. It is important to consult with a licensed chiropractor should you experience any kind of musculoskeletal pain or discomfort.

Reflexology is another form of treatment that uses pressure points in the hands, feet, and ears to stimulate healing in the body. It is based on the belief that different areas of the body are connected to specific organs and tissues. By applying gentle pressure to these points, reflexologists believe they can help unblock energy pathways and promote circulation throughout the entire body. Reflexology can be used to treat a wide range of conditions, including headaches, back pain, neck pain, and many others.

## Massage Therapists

Reflexology is a therapeutic massage technique used to alleviate pain, improve circulation, and relieve stress. It is based on the belief that there are certain areas of the feet and hands which correspond to other parts of the body. Massage therapists use specific pressure points located around these areas to create an effect within the body which can help provide relief from pain and other ailments.

The holistic approach of reflexology is one that looks at the body as a whole, recognizing the interconnectedness between each part and how this can affect overall health. Massage therapists are trained in the techniques used to help identify which areas should be targeted in order to bring relief from individual conditions. This can include gentle massage, kneading, and deeper pressure.

## What Are The Role Of Massage Therapists?

Massage therapists are responsible for evaluating and treating clients in order to help them achieve optimal health. This includes assessing the client's symptoms, performing a physical assessment, and developing a treatment plan tailored to meet their individual needs. Massage therapists can also provide preventive care by educating patients on healthy habits such as stretching and relaxation techniques that can help improve overall wellness. By combining the therapeutic effects of massage with lifestyle changes and other treatments, massage therapists can help improve their client's quality of life.

Further, massage therapists are also responsible for creating a comfortable environment in which to treat patients. This involves communicating clearly with patients about their needs and ensuring they're comfortable throughout the treatment process. It also requires an understanding of patient confidentiality in order to ensure that patients' privacy is kept.

Massage therapists are essential to the healthcare community, providing an important service for those seeking relief from pain and discomfort. By helping to reduce stress and improve circulation, massage therapy can greatly improve the quality of life for those who receive it. With proper training and knowledge, massage therapists can help create a healthier lifestyle for their clients.

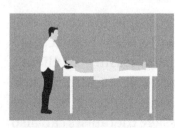

**What Is The Difference Between Acupuncturists, Naturopathic Physicians, Chiropractors, And**

## Massage Therapists?

Acupuncturists are trained in traditional Chinese medicine and use thin needles to stimulate pressure points in the body. Naturopathic physicians combine science-based natural therapies with traditional medicines to create individualized treatment plans for patients. Chiropractors specialize in treating musculoskeletal problems through hands-on manual adjustments of the spine. Massage therapists use a variety of techniques, such as Swedish massage and deep tissue massage, to alleviate physical pain and promote relaxation.

Reflexology is a holistic healing system that uses pressure points on the feet or hands to treat various health conditions in the body. Reflexologists take the time to understand their clients' needs and use specialized massage techniques to access the points to help restore balance and harmony in the body. Reflexology is often used in conjunction with other forms of natural healing, such as acupuncture and chiropractic care. It helps to improve circulation and reduce stress and muscle tension, while providing relief from pain.

When deciding which type of practitioner is right for you, it's important to consider your individual needs and preferences. For example, if you are looking to treat a specific medical condition, an acupuncturist or naturopathic physician may be more suitable than a reflexologist. On the other hand, if you are looking for relaxation and stress relief, massage therapy is often preferable. Ultimately, it's important to discuss with your practitioner which approach would be best for you.

# CONCLUSION

The earliest known history of reflexology can be traced back to Ancient Egypt, India, China and Japan. In the 5th century B.C., Egyptian medical texts describe how a physician should press certain points of the feet as part of their treatments. Meanwhile in India, Ayurvedic medicine talks about applying pressure to specific points on the hands and feet to treat various ailments. The practice of reflexology was also adopted by China and Japan, where practitioners used an ancient form of acupuncture to stimulate pressure points in the hands and feet.

Reflexology eventually became popular in Europe in the 19th century following the work of Dr William H Fitzgerald, who developed a system of 'Zone Therapy' which mapped the body into a network of ten equal vertical zones. This became popularised in the early 20th century and is still used by reflexologists today to identify which areas of the feet correspond to different parts of the body.

Today, reflexology is a widely accepted form of alternative therapy, with many practitioners offering holistic treatments based on ancient methods and modern science. It can be used as a stand-alone treatment, or combined with other forms of alternative medicine to achieve optimal results. By stimulating the feet and hands, reflexology can help to relieve stress and promote relaxation, improve circulation and stimulate the body's natural healing process.

Reflexology has become increasingly popular in recent years due to its ability to treat a wide range of physical and psychological issues. Many people use reflexology to treat conditions such as headaches, back pain, insomnia and infertility. It can also help to improve general well-being and reduce stress levels. Reflexology is now offered in many clinics, spas and health centres across the world - making it an accessible form of alternative medicine for anyone looking to achieve better physical and emotional health.

Foot Reflexology is an ancient practice that has been used in many cultures for centuries to promote wellness and healing. It is based on the idea that certain reflex points on the feet correspond to organs and systems within the body, helping to restore them back into balance. Practitioners of Reflexology believe that massaging or stimulating these reflexes can help treat a variety of ailments and conditions, from headaches to asthma.

Practitioners of Foot Reflexology use their hands, thumbs, and fingers to apply pressure to specific points on the feet. By stimulating these reflex points, they are believed to be able to reach and treat areas of the body that may be causing pain or discomfort. Additionally, Foot Reflexology is thought to help promote better circulation throughout the body and can even improve mental clarity by freeing up blocked energy pathways.

Reflexology is a gentle, non-invasive form of healing that is suitable for all ages and stages of life. It can help support the body's natural ability to heal itself and bring balance back into the body, mind, and spirit. Those who practice Reflexology often report feeling improved relaxation, and some also experience reduced pain levels, increased energy, improved sleep, and a better overall sense of well-being.

Hand Reflexology has been used for centuries to promote health and well-being. The practice involves gentle pressure applied to different points of the hands which correspond to various organs, glands, and body parts. This technique can help relieve stress, improve circulation, reduce pain and even restore balance in the body's energy system.

Today, hand reflexology is an alternative therapy increasingly being sought out by those looking to promote their physical and emotional health. It is a safe, effective treatment that can be used in conjunction with other medical treatments, as well as for preventative care. The best way to learn this practice is through taking classes or finding a certified practitioner for individual sessions.

Hand reflexology is an excellent way to focus on your overall health, allowing you to gain a greater understanding of how the body works and responds to certain treatments. It also provides an opportunity for relaxation - something that many people are in need of nowadays. With regular sessions, hand reflexology can help promote healthier habits and behaviours, resulting in improved physical and mental health.

Ear Reflexology is an ancient healing technique that was first used in the East. It works on the same principle as reflexology, which is based on the idea that certain pressure points in the body are connected to other areas of the body and can be stimulated by touching or pressing them. In-ear reflexology, specific pressure points located around the ears are targeted and treated to release blocked energy pathways and restore balance in the body.

When a practitioner performs ear reflexology, they use their fingertips to gently massage certain areas of the ears. This stimulates the corresponding parts of the brain that are connected to other organs and systems in the body. By stimulating these pressure points, practitioners aim to release tension and help improve circulation throughout the body, thus promoting better overall health and well-being.

Ear Reflexology has been used to treat a variety

of conditions, including headaches, sinus issues, anxiety, depression, fatigue and more. Recent studies have also shown that ear reflexology can be used to reduce inflammation in the body and help improve sleep quality. If you are looking for an alternative therapy to help manage stress or improve overall health and well-being, ear reflexology may be worth exploring.

Facial Reflexology is a holistic, non-invasive therapy that concentrates on specific areas of the face. It works by stimulating pressure points to activate the body's healing potential. Through this natural approach, facial reflexology can help improve overall health and well-being, as well as provide relief from stress and tension.

Facial Reflexology has been around for centuries and is based on the foundations of Chinese medicine. It works by targeting specific points on the face to provide relief from a variety of ailments. These pressure points are activated with gentle massage movements, which stimulate energy pathways throughout the body.

Facial Reflexology can help improve circulation, reduce tension headaches, and address sinus issues. It can also be used as an anti-ageing treatment as it helps to reduce wrinkles, tighten skin, and improve the overall appearance of the face. It is also a great way to de-stress and relax after a long day!

Facial Reflexology can be used in conjunction with other therapies such as massage or acupuncture for an even more holistic approach. This type of balanced approach to health and well-being is becoming increasingly popular with people looking to live a healthier life.

Auriculotherapy is a form of reflexology that focuses on the external ear. It is based on ancient Chinese medical principles and has been practiced for thousands of years. Auriculotherapy involves stimulating specific points on the ear in order to treat various physical, mental and emotional conditions. The ear contains many nerve endings, which makes it well-suited for this type of treatment. Research suggests that auriculotherapy is effective in treating a wide range of conditions, including headaches, chronic pain, depression, anxiety and even addiction.

Auriculotherapy is based on the concept that the ear acts as a micro-system for the entire body. This means that each point or area of the ear corresponds to different organs and systems of the body. Stimulating these points can help to reduce pain, improve circulation and stimulate the body's natural healing processes.

Auriculotherapy is usually performed by a trained healthcare professional such as an acupuncturist or chiropractor. During the treatment, thin needles are inserted into specific points on the ear. Depending on the condition being treated, additional forms of therapy may be used such as massage, heat or electrical stimulation.

In addition to treating physical symptoms, auriculotherapy can be used to promote relaxation and help manage stress. Stimulating certain points on the ear has been shown to induce a calming effect, which can reduce anxiety and improve mood.

## MAY I ASK YOU FOR A
## SMALL FAVOR?

Before you go, please I need your assistance! In case you like this book, might you be able to please share your opinion on Amazon and compose a legit review? It will take only one moment for you, yet be an extraordinary favour for me. Since I'm not a famous writer and I don't have a large distributing organization supporting me. I read each and every review and hop around with happiness like a little child each time my audience remark on my books and gives me their fair criticism! ☺. In case you didn't appreciate the book or had an issue with it, kindly get in touch with me via my email; d.beckology@ gmail.com and reveal to me how I can improve it.

Made in United States
Orlando, FL
30 November 2024

54687048R00104